Hormone Therapy and Cardiovascular Dynamics

W0091858

Hormone Therapy and Cardiovascular Dynamics

Carolyn Webb BSc
Clinical Physiologist and Research Assistant
Cardiac Medicine
Imperial College School of Medicine
at the National Heart & Lung Institute
London, UK

Peter Collins MD, FRCP
Senior Lecturer
& Honorary Consultant Cardiologist
Cardiac Medicine
Imperial College School of Medicine
at the National Heart & Lung Institute
and Royal Brompton Hospital
London, UK

MARTIN DUNITZ

The views expressed in this publication are
those of the authors and not necessarily those
of Martin Dunitz Ltd.

© Martin Dunitz Ltd 1997

First published in the United Kingdom
in 1997 by
Martin Dunitz Ltd
The Livery House
7– 9 Pratt Street
London NW1 0AE

A CIP record for this book is available
from the British Library.

ISBN 1-85317-409-2

Printed and bound in Spain by Cayfosa

Contents

Heart disease in women

Cardiovascular disease (CVD) is often thought of as a disease predominantly associated with men rather than women. However, CVD is currently the most common cause of death in women and is responsible for the deaths of more women than cancer, accidents and diabetes combined (Figure 1).[1] Whilst there is no basis for thinking that CVD is a disease restricted to men, there are clearly age-related differences between the two sexes. In men, the incidence of CVD increases progressively from about the age of 35, whilst in women a rapid increase is not observed until after the age of 55, and by the age of 70 the rates are almost the same.

Cardiovascular diseases are also a major cause of disability in women.[1] Not only do women present with coronary heart disease (CHD) later in life than men, but they more frequently present with angina and less frequently with sudden death. In 1980, ischaemic heart disease was assessed to be disabling in 36 per cent of women aged 55–64, and 55 per cent in women aged 75 and older.[2] The fact that CVD is as much a problem of women as of men is not always reflected in treatment patterns however. Although women experience chest pain as the main symptom of coronary artery disease more frequently than men, fewer women are referred for major diagnostic or therapeutic

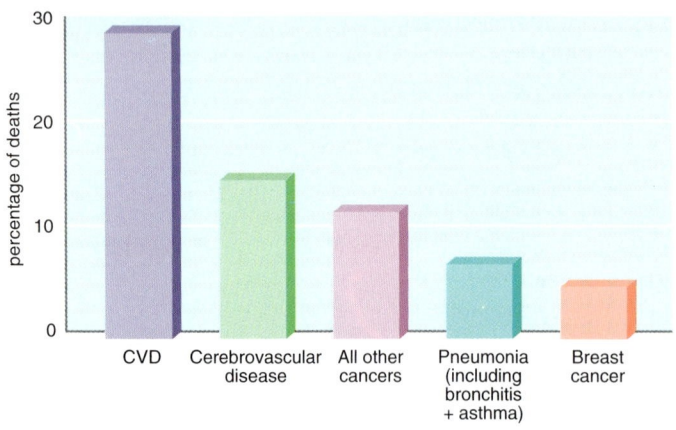

Figure 1.
Leading causes of death in UK women. [Compendium of Health Statistics, 1992 (UK data)].

tests.[3,4] Angina in women is more difficult to assess, as the diagnostic reliability of tests such as the exercise test is reduced in women; there is a greater chance of having ischaemic ECG change in the absence of significant obstructive coronary artery disease.[5] In older women with exertional angina the specificity and sensitivity of the exercise test is increased. Studies, both in Europe and North America, have shown that men with significant CHD are more likely than women to undergo revascularisation.[3-5] Although there are a number of logical factors that might explain this apparent difference,[6] some evidence suggests that despite the greater incidence of disability associated with CVD in women, physicians tend to pursue a less aggressive approach to the management and treatment of coronary disease in women as compared to men.[3]

Women have higher complication and mortality rates after myocardial infarction than men,[7-9] probably due to older age and more advanced disease. After thrombolytic therapy for myocardial infarction, women and men have similar morbidity and mortality rates, but women suffer more haemorrhagic stroke.[10] Women undergoing percutaneous transluminal coronary angioplasty (PTCA) tend to have more initial complications and a higher mortality rate than men.[11] This may be explained by a worse risk profile pre-procedure in women compared to men. Clinical success rates were comparable in men and women, as was the four-year survival rate. Women have a higher mortality rate after coronary artery bypass graft (CABG) surgery; they are older, more often diabetic and have smaller vessels for grafting.[12]

The menopause, HRT and CVD risk

Coronary heart disease

CVD rarely affects women before the menopause, strongly implicating oestrogen deficiency in the aetiology of the disease. It also suggests that naturally produced oestrogens protect women from CHD before the menopause and that therapeutic oestrogens may therefore be expected to do so after it. Support for this hypothesis comes from studies such as the Nurses Health Study which showed that the risk of coronary heart disease was more than doubled in women who have bilateral oophorectomy before the menopause, compared with women of a similar age.[13] A review of population-based case-control, cross-sectional and prospective studies of oestrogen therapy (with most using conjugated equine oestrogens) and CHD calculated the overall relative risk associated with oestrogen therapy to be reduced to 0.56.[14]

Blood pressure and hypertension

Blood pressure increases with advancing age thus confounding a precise effect of the menopause on blood pressure. There are few studies which investigate the effect of oestrogen in postmenopausal hypertensive women. Evidence from oral contraceptive users suggests an idiosyncratic detrimental effect of oestrogen therapy on blood pressure, but this is not borne out in the evidence to date. Indeed, postmenopausal oestrogen therapy appears to have a null or small beneficial effect on blood pressure. No difference in blood pressure has been observed between postmenopausal oestrogen users and non-users over a five-month period[15] and a five-year follow-up period.[16] Hazzard[17] noted that the most carefully designed studies suggested that blood pressure was consistently, although minimally, lowered by oestrogen administration.[18] The recent PEPI study showed that systolic blood pressure in the oestrogen-treated groups was not significantly different from the placebo group[19] but hypertensive subjects were not specifically enrolled in this study. A recent study[20] found no effect of hormone therapy on blood pressure in patients with hypertension who were followed up every three months for a median of fourteen months.

Stroke

Hormone therapy is not associated with increased risk of stroke and indeed there may be a protective effect.[21–30] Risk of death from stroke may also be reduced in women taking hormone therapy.[21,24,31] Grady and colleagues[32] pooled 15 studies and estimated that the relative risk for stroke from all studies was 0.96 (95 per cent CI 0.82–1.13).

Overall, the evidence strongly suggests that postmenopausal oestrogen therapy has the potential to reduce significantly the risk of CVD. The precise mode of action of this cardioprotective effect remains uncertain, but it is now known that many factors are involved, including effects on cardiovascular risk factors as well as effects directly on blood vessels (Figure 2).

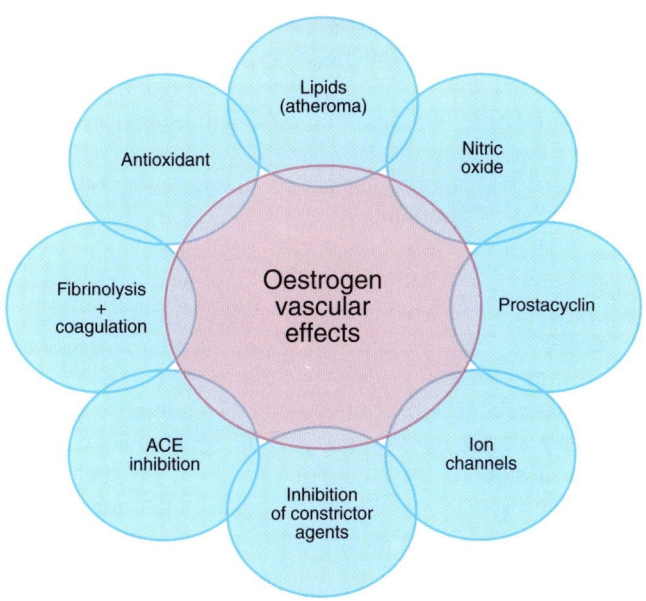

Figure 2.
Vascular effects of oestrogen. The cardioprotective effect of oestrogen is likely to involve synergism between a number of mechanisms.

Metabolic effects of postmenopausal hormone therapy

Lipids

Large-scale studies attribute 25–30 per cent of the cardioprotective effect of oestrogen to a beneficial effect on lipid profile.[14] Women aged 20–50 years have a more favourable lipid profile than men of a similar age: lower plasma low-density lipoprotein cholesterol (LDL-C) and very low-density lipoprotein (VLDL), and higher plasma high-density lipoprotein cholesterol (HDL-C). However, at the menopause there is an associated detrimental change in lipid profile, namely an increase in LDL-C and a concurrent decrease in HDL-C.[33] Oestrogen therapy reverses the negative effect of the menopause on lipids, with a particularly beneficial effect on the HDL^2 subfraction of HDL-C, which is thought to be strongly associated with cardiovascular risk. Table 1 summarises the effects of oestrogen therapy on lipid profile.

Lipid/lipoprotein	Menopause	ERT (oral)	ERT (transdermal)
LDL	↑	↓	↔or↓
HDL	↓	↑	↑
HDL^2	↓	↑	↑
Triglycerides	↑	↑	↔
Total cholesterol	↑	↓	↓

Table 1.
Summary of the effect of the menopause and oestrogen therapy on lipid profile.

Lipoprotein(a) (Lp(a)) has been suggested as an important risk factor for coronary artery disease, with high levels being associated with increased risk, as it plays an important role in removal of cholesterol from the systemic circulation.[34] Oestrogen replacement therapy in postmenopausal women lowers plasma Lp(a), as does combined oestrogen/progestogen therapy[35,36] and in this way may exert a partial beneficial effect on cardiovascular risk.

There has been concern over reports that oestrogen therapy may cause hypertriglyceridaemia;[35,37–39] however, the cardiovascular relevance of this increase is unclear. Oestrogen enhances the synthesis of VLDL triglycerides in the liver, particularly large, triglyceride-rich VLDL,[37] and since large VLDL is catabolized by the liver and is not converted to VLDL and LDL, there is possibly a less detrimental effect on cardiovascular disease risk than other triglycerides.

Insulin resistance

It is well known that diabetes is strongly associated with coronary heart disease, and diabetic women have a greater incidence of CHD than diabetic men.[40] There is a steady increase in insulin resistance with age and consequently an increase in circulating insulin concentrations. Hyperinsulinaemia may play a role in the increased risk of cardiovascular disease in postmenopausal women. Changes in glucose and insulin metabolism in postmenopausal women may be implicated in the changes in lipid profile associated with the menopause and the predisposition to coronary heart disease in women after the menopause. Hormone replacement therapy has a beneficial effect on insulin resistance by increasing insulin clearance, thus preventing hyperinsulinaemia associated with insulin resistance.[41,42]

Body fat

Obesity is a risk factor for cardiovascular disease, but it is the distribution of body fat rather than total body fat which is of particular relevance to cardiovascular disease risk. Premenopausal women tend to have a peripheral (gynoid) body fat distribution, whilst central (android) fat distribution (associated with increased risk of coronary heart disease) is found predominantly in postmenopausal women and men.[43] HRT prevents increases in abdominal fat and redistributes to a favourable gynoid fat distribution independent of serum lipids or lipoproteins, with little effect on total body fat.[44]

Haemostasis

Recent evidence suggests a statistically significant, but probably biologically less significant, increase in the incidence of venous thromboembolus[45,46] and pulmonary embolus[47] in current users of postmenopausal hormone therapy. Daly et al[45] found no difference in venous thromboembolus incidence in women taking either oestrogen alone or combination oestrogen and progestogen, oral versus transdermal route of administration, or high or low oestrogen dose. In contrast, a population-based study found a significant increase in venous thromboembolus with increasing oestrogen dose in postmenopausal conjugated oestrogen users.[46] For current users versus non-users of oestrogen, a dose of 0.325 mg daily was associated with a relative risk of 2.1, whereas 0.625 mg and 1.25 mg was associated with a relative risk of 3.3 and 6.9 respectively (95 per cent. CI). A dose of 1.25 mg daily of conjugated oestrogen is rarely used nowadays, however.

Recent evidence suggests that a reduction in plasma fibrinolytic activity may be a marker for an increased risk of cardiovascular disease. Markers of endogenous fibrinolysis, such as levels of tissue-type plasminogen activator (TPA) antigen and plasminogen activator inhibitor-1 (PAI-1), have been associated with an increased risk of cardiovascular diseases such as coronary heart disease, myocardial infarction, thrombosis and stroke. The menopause has a tendency to affect haemostatic variables adversely. The procoagulant factor VII levels increase[48] as do plasma fibrinogen[49] and tissue plasminogen activator levels, indicating an increased risk of arterial thrombosis due to hypercoagulability. PAI-1, a factor which is negatively related to fibrinolysis, is elevated in postmenopausal women.[50]

Observational studies have shown a beneficial effect of hormone therapy on endogenous fibrinolytic activity, reporting higher levels of plasminogen or lower levels of PAI-1 and/or

TPA antigens.[51] These data indicate an enhanced fibrinolytic potential in current users of hormone therapy compared with non-users. Other smaller studies have found no association between oestrogen therapy and venous thrombosis[52] or thromboembolism.[53]

Vascular responses to oestrogen

There is now evidence to support the presence of direct vascular effects of oestrogen, which in turn support the biological plausibility of the epidemiological findings of cardioprotection in oestrogen users, and may also explain the effect of acutely and chronically administered oestrogen on blood flow.

Blood flow

Coronary circulation — direct vascular smooth muscle effects

Oestrogen induces dilatation of conductance and resistance coronary arteries, albeit at supraphysiologic concentrations (>0.1 µmol/l), in dogs when administered acutely into the coronary circulation.[54] By removing the endothelium and using inhibitors of adenosine triphosphate-sensitive potassium and calcium channels, it was shown that this effect is endothelium-independent and is mediated by effects on adenosine triphosphate-sensitive potassium and/or calcium channels. Experiments using a classic intracellular oestrogen receptor antagonist showed that the receptor is not involved in the response.

Coronary circulation — indirect, endothelium-dependent effects

In ovariectomized animals, long-term (two years)[55] oestrogen replacement therapy reverses acetylcholine (ACh)-induced constriction in atherosclerotic coronary arteries, and a similar effect is produced with a 20-minute intravenous infusion of ethinyl oestradiol.[56] These animal data have been reproduced in postmenopausal women with coronary atherosclerosis. Oestrogen attenuates[57] or abolishes[58,59] ACh-induced vasoconstriction when administered acutely (15–20 minutes after bolus or continuous intracoronary infusion) in these women, resulting in increased coronary diameter and flow. This response of the coronary arteries to ACh after exposure to 17β-oestradiol appears to be gender-dependent.[59] A 20-minute exposure to 17β-oestradiol modulated ACh-induced responses of female but not male atherosclerotic coronary arteries *in vivo* (Figure 3). Current, chronic, physiological oestrogen replacement has also been shown to influence endothelium-dependent and independent coronary responsiveness to ACh.[60] Oestrogen replacement therapy was associated with an attenuation or reversal of the coronary vasoconstrictor response to ACh in postmenopausal women. This suggests a possible normalization of an endothelium-dependent mechanism in diseased coronary vessels, in agreement with the effect of acutely administered oestrogen. Such an effect could contribute to an oestrogen-induced reduction in cardiovascular events associated with oestrogen therapy.

Peripheral circulation — probable direct vascular smooth muscle effects

In the oestrogen-deplete state, local and systemic administration of 17β-oestradiol has actions on both reproductive and non-reproductive vascular beds.[61] The effect of oestrogen administration on systemic haemodynamics has been studied in postmenopausal women. Forty minutes after the administration of sublingual 17β-oestradiol to postmenopausal volunteers

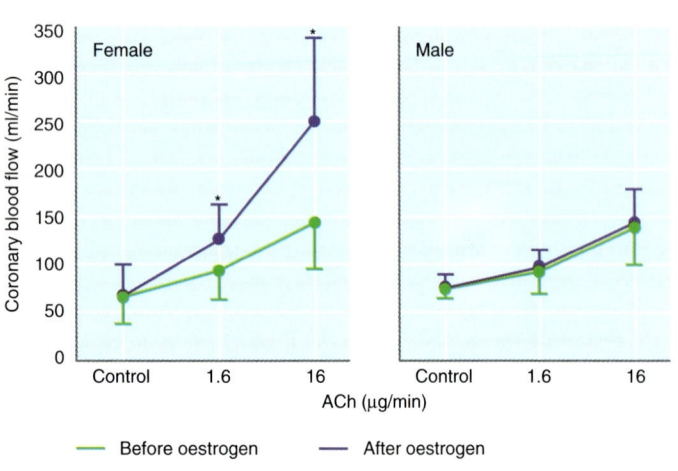

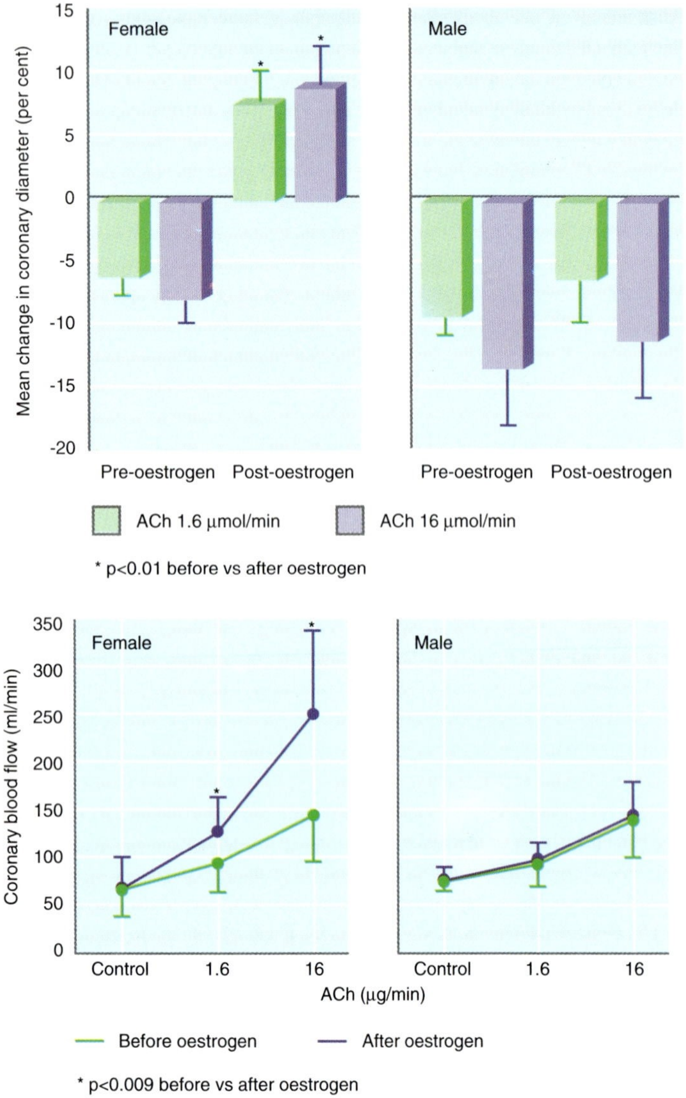

Figure 3.
*Acute oestrogen administration reverses ACh-induced vasoconstriction and increases blood flow in human female, but not male, coronary arteries (*Circulation *1995; **92**: 24-30).*

there was an increase in forearm blood flow and a reduction in forearm vascular resistance compared to placebo, with no difference in mean arterial blood pressure (Figure 4).[62] Relatively high plasma levels of 17β-oestradiol (≈3000 pmol per litre)

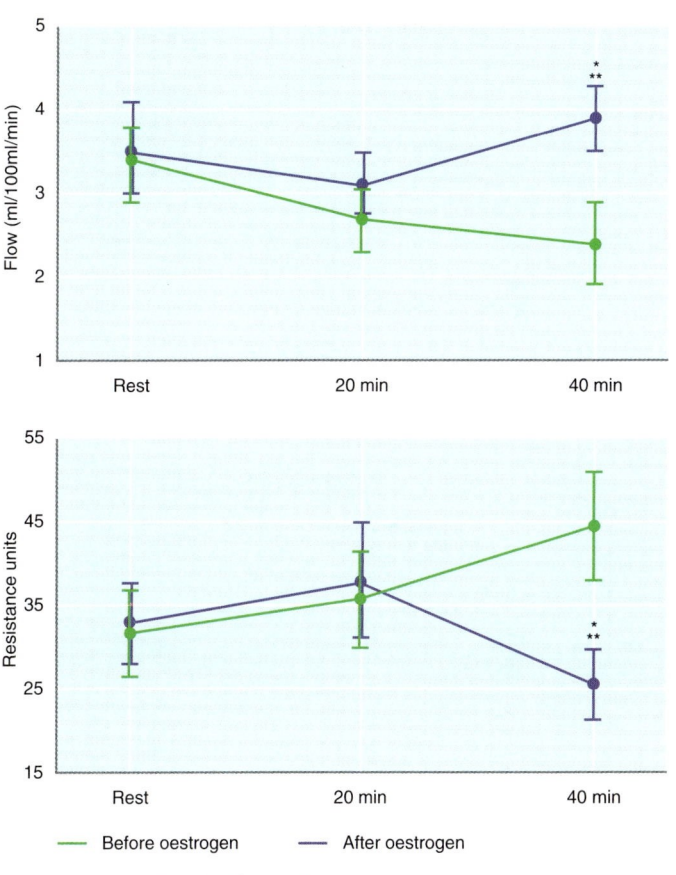

— Before oestrogen — After oestrogen

* p<0.05 oestradiol-17β 20 vs 40 minutes
** p<0.05 oestradiol-17β vs placebo at 40 minutes

Figure 4.
Acute sublingual oestrogen administration in postmenopausal women increases forearm blood flow and decreases forearm vascular resistance (Am J Med 1995; 99: 119-122).

were achieved in these women (midcycle level ≈1800 pmol per litre). However the plasma levels were approximately 50 per cent of those found in pregnancy. Similar changes in blood flow have been demonstrated in the blood supply to the leg.[63]

Peripheral circulation — endothelium-dependent effects

The role of endogenous ovarian hormones in modulating peripheral vasoreactivity has recently been investigated in pre-menopausal women.[64] Endothelium-dependent vasodilatation, induced by hyperaemia, varied significantly with the phase of the menstrual cycle, with flow-mediated increases in brachial artery diameter being less during the menstrual phase of the cycle (when serum oestradiol levels were low), than in the fol-licular or luteal phase of the cycle (when serum oestradiol levels were elevated) (Figure 5). This suggests that endoge-nous oestradiol may be involved in the mediation of variations

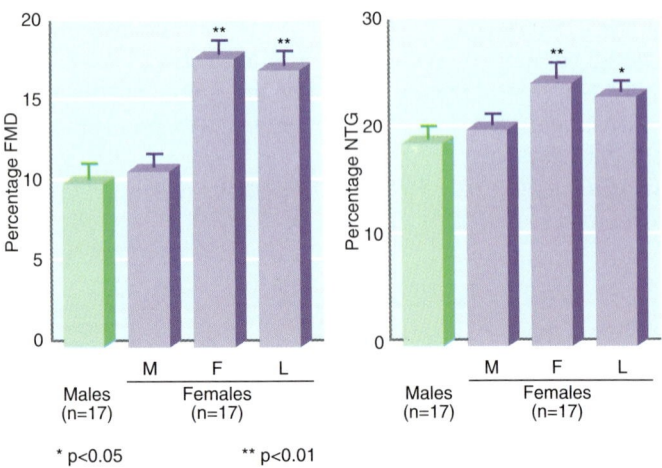

Figure 5.
Effects of sex and menstrual cycle on flow-mediated diameter (FMD) of the brachial artery. Percentage increases in artery diameter induced by hyperaemia and glyceryl trinitrate (NTG) (Circulation 1995; 92: 3431-3435).

in endothelium-dependent brachial artery with the menstrual cycle. It also emphasizes an effect of ovarian hormones at physiological plasma levels and confirms similar findings with oestrogen treatment.

In postmenopausal women forearm vasodilatation induced by ACh is potentiated by the acute local administration of intravenous oestradiol,[65] suggesting that endothelium-dependent responses in the peripheral circulation may be modulated by steroid hormones *in vivo* in humans. Oestrogen increases flow-mediated vasodilatation in the brachial artery of postmenopausal women.[66] Decreases in arterial waveform pulsatility index (PI) in the uterine and carotid arteries have been observed in postmenopausal women after chronic oestrogen therapy.[67] An increased PI is closely correlated with the time elapsed after the menopause, and this increase is thought to indicate a reduction in arterial compliance, and therefore could reflect a decrease in blood flow. Oestrogen therapy reverses increased pulsatility index, suggesting an improvement in arterial compliance.

The acute effect of oestrogen on forearm blood flow may be mediated, at least in part, by the calcium antagonistic property of oestrogen resulting in vascular myocyte relaxation and arterial dilatation. Longer-term effects on blood flow may involve the nitric oxide (NO) pathway and may be oestrogen-receptor dependent.

New and unexpected mechanisms of oestrogen on the vessel wall have been discovered in recent years which support the hypothesis that oestrogen has an important role in vascular homeostasis in women. Although the magnitude of the benefits of oestrogen on the vascular system are not fully evaluated, the evidence suggests that these mechanisms have clinical relevance to cardiovascular physiology and pathophysiology.

Oestrogen receptor

Receptor-dependent mechanisms are involved in the response of blood vessels of the reproductive system to gonadal hormones, and oestrogen receptors are found in a number of other tissues including the heart and liver.[68,69] Recent data suggest that the acute effects of oestrogen in other circulations may be independent of the classical oestrogen receptor. Receptor-dependent mechanisms may be involved in chronic vascular effects, but there are no data which prove this hypothesis. There are conflicting data on the presence of oestrogen receptors in female human coronary arteries. They have been demonstrated in normal coronary arteries but there is variable expression in atherosclerotic coronary arteries from premenopausal women.[70] Others have found no evidence for oestrogen receptors in normal coronary arteries, using a different antibody technique.[71] Recent studies using specific monoclonal antibodies and nuclear probes have confirmed the presence of a classical oestrogen receptor in cultured human umbilical, aortic and coronary artery endothelial cells,[72,73] suggesting that the cardioprotective effect of oestrogen may, at least in part, be due to effects on endothelial cell function via the oestrogen receptor. A novel oestrogen receptor has recently been cloned in rat prostate, called oestrogen-receptor-beta, or ER-β.[74] This receptor was also found in the ovary and had high affinity to 17β-oestradiol. At present no such receptor has been identified in human tissue, but this finding raises the possibility of cardiac or/and vascular-specific oestrogen receptors which may be involved in the modulation of vascular responses to oestrogen.

Endothelium/nitric oxide-mediated effects

The endothelium has been shown to mediate the relaxing effect to 17β-oestradiol in isolated vessels from animals. Increased endothelium-dependent relaxation to ACh and attenuation of the development of hypertension has been demonstrated in oestrogen-treated spontaneously hypertensive rat aorta.[75] Femoral arteries treated with 17β-oestradiol show an enhanced endothelium-dependent relaxation to ACh at small concentrations.[76] These data have been confirmed in postmenopausal women where forearm vasodilatation induced by ACh is potentiated by the acute local administration of intravenous oestradiol[65] suggesting that endothelium-dependent responses may be modulated by steroid hormones.

Nitric oxide

Nitric oxide (NO) causes vasorelaxation in endothelium-intact coronary arteries and is a product of the conversion of L-arginine by NO synthases (NOS) to NO and citrulline. NOS can be divided into two functional groups based on their calcium sensitivity. Oestrogen can induce calcium-dependent NOS, thus enhancing the amount of available NOS in a cell.[77] NO has also been observed to slow the development of atheroma by inhibiting smooth muscle cell proliferation while stimulating proliferation of endothelial cells.[78] Oestrogen is a potent antioxidant of lipids[79] and oxidized lipids inhibit NO.[80] Oestrogen may therefore protect the vasculature via enhanced NO production or by prolonging the half life of released NO which in turn has antiatherogenic properties. The time course for this effect is unknown and may be relevant only with long-term oestrogen treatment. An increased basal release of NO in endothelium-intact aortic rings from female rabbits than those from males has been reported.[81] Oestrogen-induced nitric oxide effects on vascular protection are summarized in Figure 6.

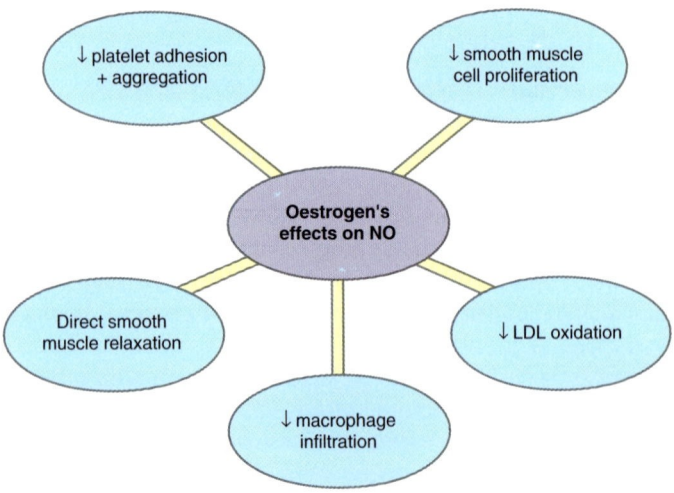

Figure 6.
Oestrogen-induced nitric oxide effects on vascular protection.

The sex hormone status of the animal may be important in determining whether NO plays a role in the oestrogen-induced coronary and basilar artery relaxation.[82–84] Female rabbits which were oestrogen-treated and then acutely oestrogen with-drawn (mimicking a perimenopausal state) demonstrated an increased sensitivity to the relaxing effect of 17β-oestradiol, which was found to be endothelium- and NO-dependent. Oestrogen-induced, endothelium-dependent relaxation of coronary arteries may therefore, in some species, depend on the sex hormone status of the animal.

A recent study in humans has demonstrated a variation in expired NO production with cyclical hormone changes in pre-menopausal women, with NO levels peaking at the middle of the menstrual cycle[85] suggesting an influence of gonadal hormones on the synthesis and release of NO in humans.

Nitric oxide synthase

Oestrogen can stimulate constitutive NOS in cultured endothelial cells[86] and in tissues from oestrogen-treated animals,[77] an effect which takes many hours or even days to become apparent. Recent experiments in cultured human umbilical vein endothelial cells show that oestrogen stimulates basal NOS six-fold within 30 minutes in human tissue.[87] An oestrogen-induced increase of coronary flow in isolated hearts from ovariectomized female animals was abolished by NOS inhibition,[88] as was oestrogen-induced uterine vasodilatation in ewes.[89]

Sex hormones have effects on calcium-dependent NO production and protein levels of NOS in cultured human aortic endothelial cells. Endothelial and NO stimulation was shown to occur at physiological concentrations of 17β-oestradiol.[90] Recent data demonstrate increased endothelial-derived NO activity and increased NOS messenger RNA in pregnancy in rats;[91] an effect which was attributable to oestrogen. These data strongly suggest that human endothelium and NOS can be regulated by oestrogens.

Calcium antagonistic effect

Endothelium-independent vasorelaxation has been demon-strated *in vitro* in animal and human coronary arteries[92,93] suggesting an action of oestrogen directly on vascular smooth muscle cells. Calcium antagonistic properties of oestrogen have been observed in uterine arteries and in isolated smooth muscle cells from uterine arteries and veins.[94] 17β-oestradiol has similar relaxing effects on contraction induced by activation of both receptor-operated and potential-operated calcium chan-nels in rabbit coronary arteries.[92] A calcium antagonist effect of 17β-oestradiol has been confirmed in isolated guinea pig myocytes using electrophysiological and calcium indicator studies, showing a decrease in calcium current and intracellu-lar levels of calcium in these cells. These experiments proved that oestrogen was acting as a calcium antagonist at the con-centrations used (Figure 7).[95]

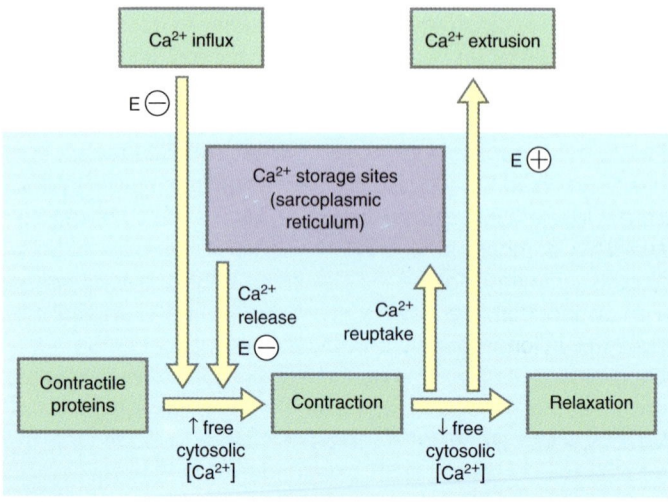

Figure 7.
Vascular smooth muscle relaxation by oestrogen-induced effects on calcium ion movement. Oestrogen inhibits the influx of calcium across the plasma membrane and inhibits the release of calcium from the sarcoplasmic reticulum. These mechanisms result in a decrease in free cytosolic calcium levels and lead to smooth muscle relaxation. E- = inhibition by oestrogen, E+ = enhancement by oestrogen.

Oestrogen can inhibit the contraction of epicardial coronary arteries by inhibiting calcium influx without changing calcium sensitivity of contractile elements (Figure 7).[96] Further evidence that 17β-oestradiol has effects on calcium channels in vascular smooth muscle cells is provided by work on an isolated vascular smooth muscle cell line (A7r5) using whole patch-clamp techniques.[97] 17β-oestradiol significantly reduced L-type barium currents and T-type calcium currents within 1–2 minutes. This was in contrast to 17α-oestradiol, which caused significantly less reduction in both types of current. The calcium antagonistic effect of oestrogen may be involved in its inhibitory effect on vascular smooth muscle cell proliferation. Most of the acute effects in vascular smooth muscle cells occur at micromolar concentrations which are three to four orders of magnitude greater than achieved in the normal female circulatory system. However, it is possible that tissues accumulate lipid soluble steroids and local concentrations could theoretically reach this level.

As well as effects on calcium channels, oestrogen affects large conductance chloride channels by a direct membrane effect.[98] These channels, in cultured fibroblasts, were inhibited by exposure to extracellular, but not intracellular, anti-oestrogen, and this effect could be prevented by extracellular 17β-oestradiol, but not intracellular 17β-oestradiol or extracellular 17β-oestradiol. This demonstrates another regulatory role for ovarian steroids, affecting plasma ion channels via membrane binding sites distinct from the classical oestrogen receptor and subsequent activation of intracellular second-messenger pathway(s).

Modulation of neurotransmission

Oestrogen modulates the sympathetic and parasympathetic autonomic nervous systems. Oestrogen inhibits the activity of tyrosine hydroxylase which synthesizes catecholamines through feedback inhibition after being converted to catechol oestrogen.[99] Release of noradrenaline during sympathetic activation is modified by noradrenaline stimulation of α_2-adrenoceptors. Oestrogen increases the density and enhances the function of α_2-adrenoceptors[100] and attenuates sympathetic activity.

Postmenopausal women have increased basal levels of plasma noradrenaline compared with premenopausal women. They also have an elevated stress-induced increase in plasma noradrenaline concentrations.[101] These increased pressor and neurohormonal responses in postmenopausal women are partially inhibited by oestrogen.[101] The inhibitory effect of oestrogen on noradrenaline synthesis may have a long-term beneficial effect on atherogenesis, since increased sympathetic activity is associated with atheroma development.[102] Hyperadrenergic states increase vascular smooth muscle proliferation, increase vascular permeability to calcium and increase vascular permeability to lipoproteins, all of which can enhance the tendency to develop atheroma.

The activity of the cholinergic-muscarinic system in the central nervous system is potentiated by oestrogen.[103] The content of ACh and the activity of choline acetyltransferase is increased in females when compared to males,[103] is reduced after oophorectomy[104] and is increased by subsequent oestrogen treatment.[103] Choline uptake is increased by oestrogen and decreased after oophorectomy.[105] Greater parasympathetic activity in normal women compared to men has been demonstrated by measurement of heart rate variability.[106]

The balance of these two systems in the oestrogen-deficient postmenopausal woman is in favour of sympathetic overactivity, which could result in both atheroma development and a tendency to an increase in acute vascular events. A normalization of sympathetic activity may therefore contribute to oestrogen's protective effect on the cardiovascular system in postmenopausal women.

Renin–angiotensin system

Experiments in resistance vessels show that they have the capacity to generate angiotensin II from renin substrate, and the effect can be blocked by specific renin inhibitors.[107] Vascular renin may influence local vessel tone in a number of ways. Angiotensin II produced locally could constrict vascular smooth muscle directly. It may also modulate peripheral sympathetic neurotransmission, increasing sympathetic activity.[108] Locally released angiotensin II can act as a vascular growth factor.[109] Angiotensin-converting enzyme has been identified on the luminal surface of the vascular endothelium[110] and in the media and adventitia of blood vessels.[111]

Oestrogen inhibits angiotensin II-induced constrictor effects both *in vitro* and *in vivo*.[112,113] In addition, it has recently been shown that oestrogen has angiotensin-converting enzyme inhibitor properties in postmenopausal women.[114] This mechanism could be involved in long-term vascular protection by inhibiting the influence of the vasoconstrictor angiotensin II and possible enhancement of NO synthesis. Inhibition of the angiotensin-converting enzyme by oestrogen may increase tissue levels of bradykinin (which is also broken down by the enzyme) which, in turn, stimulates the release of NO and vasodilating prostaglandins.[115,116]

Endothelin-1

Oestrogen inhibits the constrictor responses to endothelin-1 in rabbit coronary arteries.[117] Plasma endothelin-1 levels increase following ACh infusion in pigs with coronary atheroma[118] and although this has not yet been confirmed in humans, it may suggest that the reversal of the constrictor effect of ACh in human atherosclerotic coronary arteries *in vivo* by oestrogen[57–59] may be partially explained by oestrogen-induced inhibition of endothelin-1-induced contraction.

Prostacyclin

Prostacyclin (PGI_2) is a prostaglandin produced by the endothelial cells and its synthesis is coupled to EDRF release.[119] It can induce vasodilatation and inhibition of platelet activation. Oestrogen can upregulate the production of prostacyclin.[120] Chang et al[121] demonstrated an enhancement of basal levels of prostacyclin secretion in rat aortic smooth muscle cells exposed to oestradiol. This was thought to be mediated via an increase in transcription of genes for the enzymes prostacyclin synthetase and prostaglandin cyclo-oxygenase. The evidence is scant, however, and has yet to be demonstrated in human tissue, but there is an indication that oestrogen may affect coagulation and vasorelaxation by its effects on prostacyclin, since NO and prostacyclin have been shown to modulate favourably monocyte-vascular wall interactions.[122]

Acute events

Oestrogen has been shown to affect a number of regulatory mechanisms, resulting in a tendency towards a state of vascular relaxation. The resulting decrease of vascular shear stress forces has the potential to protect vascular beds from long-term damage. This could lead to a reduction in the development of atheroma and the tendency of atherosclerotic plaque rupture, resulting in fewer acute cardiovascular events such as myocardial infarction and stroke.

Thrombogenesis

The effect of oestrogen on acute vascular reactivity may be relevant to the onset of acute events, and possibly the prevention of acute events by preserving normal endothelial function and therefore decreasing the tendency to vasoconstriction and plaque rupture. Experimental and clinical studies have shown that the endothelium, in the presence of risk factors, loses the ability to produce the vasodilator NO and therefore may be involved in the genesis of atherosclerosis and may enhance a tendency to vasoconstriction.[123–125]

Oestrogen's effects on haemostatic factors (discussed earlier), favouring a tendency towards fibrinolysis[51] do not support the widely held belief that treatment of postmenopausal women with oestrogen increases arterial thrombotic tendency. In contrast, accompanied by the favourable effect of hormone therapy on platelet aggregability, these data may explain, in part, the favourable association of hormone therapy with cardiovascular disease risk.

The picture may be different for venous thrombosis. Recent data suggest a slight increase in the tendency to venous thrombosis in low-risk postmenopausal women taking hormone therapy (5 per 100,000 woman years).[47] This adverse risk which is not accompanied by an increased mortality would appear to be far outweighed by the potential benefit on overall cardiovascular disease risk.

Platelets

Platelet activity is influenced by hormonal status and hormone treatment. 17β-oestradiol reduces platelet adherence to the endothelium *in vitro*.[126] Platelet aggregability is reduced by oestrogen which may be due to an inhibitory effect on calcium handling in human platelets.[127] Platelet aggregation is also reduced in postmenopausal women after oestrogen treatment.[128]

NO can inhibit monocyte adhesion,[122] synthesize factors which enhance chemotaxis of monocytes[129] and reduce platelet aggregation.[130] This 'indirect' mechanism may synergize with the 'direct' effects of oestrogen on platelet function to reduce platelet aggregation and thus thrombotic tendency.

Prostacyclin

Oestrogen's effects on prostacyclin and on haemostatic profile suggest that postmenopausal oestrogen therapy may decrease acute vascular events like myocardial infarction and stroke by decreasing thrombus formation. The enhanced release or prolongation of activity of NO by oestrogen, possibly via effects on NOS, may also protect against the evolution of acute vascular events by decreasing vascular shear-stress forces. These hypotheses, however, have not been proven.

Myocardial infarction

A tendency towards an increase in thrombolysis and a decrease in platelet aggregability by oestrogen could contribute to a decreased tendency to acute vascular events. Oestrogen therapy reduces the risk of myocardial infarction in post-menopausal women.[21,131-133] The risk of myocardial infarction is also decreased in high-risk women with a previous history of cardiovascular disease or myocardial infarction.[21,29,131,134] It is plausible that the vasorelaxant effect of oestrogen on the coronary arteries, coupled with a tendency towards a decrease in thrombosis, may be major contributory factors resulting in a decrease in acute cardiovascular events such as myocardial infarction.

Chronic disease processes — atherosclerosis

The fact that postmenopausal oestrogen supplementation appears to decrease death from myocardial infarction, stroke and cardiovascular disease in general, supports the concept that it has beneficial effects on the atherosclerotic process. Retrospective angiographic studies show a protective effect of oestrogen on atheroma progression in humans. Oestrogen users have less coronary artery occlusion compared to non-users[135] and less angiographically significant coronary artery disease,[136] an effect which is independent of the type of menopause or other cardiovascular risk factors, except high-density lipoprotein (HDL) cholesterol. Oestrogen has beneficial effects on a variety of factors involved in the atherogenic process which may explain these clinical findings.

Long-term calcium antagonist treatment is known to decrease the progression of atheroma when given to patients with established coronary heart disease.[137,138] It has been hypothesized that some of the cardiovascular benefit of oestrogen replacement therapy may be due to the calcium antagonist effect of oestrogen.[139] In a long-term study of oestrogen in ovariectomized, high cholesterol fed cynomolgus monkeys, a decrease in coronary atheroma was reported compared to the non-treated animals.[140] Similar findings have been demonstrated in humans in an angiographic study of postmenopausal oestrogen users.[136] Calcium antagonists have not been shown to affect outcome, however; therefore the precise clinical relevance of the calcium antagonist property of oestrogen has yet to be fully determined.

Oestrogen increases the synthesis and/or prolongs the half-life of NO, and it is a powerful antioxidant of lipids. Oxidized lipids inhibit NO. Oestrogen may beneficially affect atherogenesis via these effects on NO.

The inhibitory effect of oestrogen on norepinephrin synthesis may have a long-term beneficial effect on atherogenesis, since increased sympathetic activity is associated with atheroma development.[102] Hyperadrenergic states increase vascular smooth muscle proliferation, increase vascular permeability to calcium and increase vascular permeability to lipoproteins—all of which can enhance atheroma development.

Plaque formation

Lipids

Details of changes at the menopause and effects of postmenopausal oestrogen therapy on lipid profile have been discussed earlier. Coronary atherosclerotic plaque size is decreased in animals treated with long-term oestrogen replacement.[141] The mechanism of this effect may be due in part to either a decrease in the uptake of LDL into the arterial wall and/or an increase in the degradation of LDL in the arterial wall.

Antioxidant properties

Antioxidants have the ability to restore endothelium-dependent vasodilatation in atherosclerotic vessels. Atherosclerosis impairs endothelium-dependent vasodilatation and this is positively related to the production of oxygen-derived free radicals.[142] Free radicals can inactivate NO by direct combination at the vascular wall site. They can also damage the endothelium by oxidizing LDL particles which results in impairment of the endothelium to produce NO.[143] Oestrogen may therefore be antiatherogenic via enhanced NO production or protection from NO degradation.

Peroxidation of LDL greatly increases its atherogenicity[79] and the oxidation products have various effects which may promote plaque progression and instability.[144] Oestrogen is a potent antioxidant of lipids,[79] an effect which may be related to the phenolic ring in its structure.[145] It has been shown in hypercholesterolaemic animals that 17β-oestradiol can preserve endothelial vasodilator function and limit LDL oxidation. The susceptibility of LDL to oxidation is also reduced in postmenopausal women who have been treated with oestrogen when administered both acutely and for three weeks.[79] This antioxidant effect of oestrogen may have anti-atherogenic implications by decreasing LDL oxidation, foam cell formation and accumulation of lipid within the vessel wall.

Smooth muscle cell proliferation

The vascular endothelium provides a metabolic surface that is vasodilatory, anticoagulant and anti-adhesive for leucocytes and also inhibits proliferation of vascular smooth muscle cells.[123] NO can slow the development of atheroma by inhibiting smooth cell proliferation while stimulating proliferation of endothelial cells.[78] Oestrogen may have a beneficial effect on smooth muscle cell proliferation via its ability to induce NOS, and enhance levels of NO or prolong its half-life. Proliferation of vascular smooth muscle cells in culture is inhibited by 17β-oestradiol.[146] These *in vitro* findings may have important, as yet undetermined, implications on atheroma development in humans. Preliminary reports suggest it may be able to inhibit the restenosis phenomenon after balloon coronary angioplasty.[147]

Vessel wall structure

Oestrogen has been shown to affect the extracellular matrix of the vessel wall, which may contribute to plaque stability.[148] Oestrogen alters the proportion of collagen and elastin in the vessel wall, enhancing the ratio of procollagen type 1 to procollagen type 3, for example;[149,150] this may result in increased plaque stability. In theory the relative rate of turnover and accumulation of collagen and elastin could affect the stiffness of the wall and therefore may be implicated in the development of pathology of the vessel. Oestrogen has the potential to enhance the development of the collateral coronary circulation in the presence of flow-limiting stenoses. *In vitro* work suggests that oestrogen can enhance the migration and proliferation of endothelial cells facilitating the organization into tubular networks which may be critical to angiogenesis,[151] a response which may limit myocardial damage should abrupt thrombotic closure of a coronary vessel occur.

Relevance of vascular effects
of oestrogen to potential
therapeutic option for CVD

Myocardial ischaemia

Oestrogen-induced reduction in vascular resistance and increases in coronary flow may have clinical implications with regard to exercise-induced myocardial ischaemia, where coronary stenoses may become flow limiting. Rosano et al[152] demonstrated a beneficial effect of acute administration of sublingual 17β-oestradiol versus placebo on signs of exercise-induced myocardial ischaemia on the electrocardiogram (time to 1 mm ST-segment depression) and exercise tolerance in postmenopausal women. Patients with low plasma 17β-oestradiol levels generally had a greater response to 17β-oestradiol. Plasma levels achieved in this study were of the order of 2500 pmol per litre, which is above the peak level found at mid-cycle (midcycle level ≈1800 pmol per litre) and about one third of the level found in pregnancy. This effect may be due to a direct relaxing effect on the coronary arteries,[93] peripheral vasodilatation,[62] or a combination of the two. Further studies will be required to prove the efficacy of oestrogen therapy in the treatment of angina in the presence of coronary artery disease.

Hypertension

A decrease in peripheral vascular resistance induced by oestrogen, via endothelium-dependent and independent effects, would indicate that there may be a possible beneficial effect of oestrogen in patients with hypertension. Endothelium-dependent vasorelaxation is decreased in patients with essential hypertension.[153] Oestrogen may confer a similar benefit to patients with essential hypertension via its effects on the endothelium and NO, favouring endothelium-dependent vasorelaxation[66] and also possibly via its calcium antagonist property in vascular smooth muscle.[96] The recently discovered angiotensin-converting enzyme inhibitor effect of oestrogen[114] may have exciting implications in the treatment of hypertension (and possibly heart failure), but there is no clinical evidence to support this hypothesis as yet.

Cardiological syndrome X

Angina pectoris is usually caused by obstructive atheromatous coronary artery disease, but angiographically smooth coronary arteries are found in approximately 20 per cent of patients who undergo coronary angiography[154] and the majority of these patients are women. The triad of angina pectoris, a positive exercise test and angiographically smooth coronary arteries is commonly referred to as syndrome X, a term first used by Kemp et al in 1973.[155] The pathophysiology of the troublesome chest pain in syndrome X is poorly understood, and there are many suggested mechanisms.[156–158] Although syndrome X is likely to be a heterogeneous condition, reduced coronary flow reserve induced by dipyridamole has been reported in many patients with this diagnosis.[157,159] Most of the women with syndrome X are postmenopausal[160] and a recent study which investigated the clinical and gynaecological features of female patients with syndrome X found that ovarian hormone deficiency played a role in unmasking the syndrome in female patients.[161] Oestrogen therapy may be helpful in the treatment of this condition by decreasing the occurrence of chest pain.[162] There was no effect on exercise tolerance, which may be related to the fact that only a small number of patients with syndrome X suffer true myocardial ischaemia.

Supraventricular tachycardia

A recent study in healthy premenopausal women showed cyclical variation in the occurrence of paroxysmal supraventricular tachycardia (SVT) with the menstrual cycle, and a relationship between ovarian hormones and paroxysmal SVT.[163] An increased incidence of SVT was found during the luteal phase of the menstrual cycle which may be linked to increased sympathetic activity. This could be a result of decreased oestrogen levels and/or increased progesterone levels. Electrophysiological effects of oestrogen on the heart are relatively unexplored however.

Conclusions

Heart disease is as common in women as in men, but it occurs in women later in life. The menopause, and its associated oestrogen deficiency, appear to be risk factors for the development of cardiovascular disease in women, and post-menopausal oestrogen therapy has been shown to decrease this risk. The mechanisms involved include effects on metabolism, plasma lipids in particular, as well as effects on vascular physiology and pathophysiology. Oestrogen decreases vascular tone by a number of different mechanisms including endothelium-derived nitric oxide and prostanoids, ion channel modulation, inhibition of constrictor factors and others.

Advantageous effects on acute and chronic blood flow by oestrogen may also involve these mechanisms, and they may at least partially account for the beneficial effects of oestrogen on atherogenesis.

Until recently, cardiovascular disease was a contraindication for patients receiving postmenopausal hormone therapy. Certainly this is now not the case and indeed there is a strong argument for the use of oestrogen in the prevention of cardio-vascular disease.

Vascular effects of progestogens

Epidemiological evidence

Non-hysterectomized women who take postmenopausal hormone therapy take a cyclical or continuous progestogen in combination with oestrogen to protect against uterine cancer. Progesterone is an antagonist of oestrogen in the reproductive system, and it is assumed, therefore, that the addition of a progestogen opposes the beneficial effects of oestrogen on the cardiovascular system. The cardioprotective effects of oestrogen replacement therapy do not seem to be attenuated when combined with a progestogen, and indeed a reduction in risk has been demonstrated.[25,27,133,164–167] Studies investigating the effect of combination oestrogen and progestogen therapy on the risk of myocardial infarction showed similar protective effects to oestrogens alone,[133,166] although these studies were too small to produce statistically significant results. Oestrogen combined with a cyclical progestogen (500 µg norgestrel for ten days) decreased the relative risk of first acute myocardial infarction by 50 per cent.[133] Combination therapy also had little effect on the beneficial effect of oestrogen therapy on mortality in women with established coronary heart disease in another study.[32] A recent evaluation of the Nurses Health Study population has shown no detrimental effect of a progestin added to oestrogen therapy on cardiovascular disease risk.[168]

Combination therapy also has no increase in the risk of stroke.[25,164] The epidemiological evidence may be partially explained by effects on lipid profile.[35,36]

Scientific evidence

Jiang et al[169] examined the direct effect of progesterone on rabbit coronary arteries and aorta in vitro, and demonstrated endothelium-independent relaxation to progesterone, indicating that progesterone may have different effects on the reproductive and cardiovascular circulations. In endothelium-denuded coronary arteries, progesterone shifted calcium concentration-dependent constrictor-response curves to the right, and the maximal contraction was also reduced, indicating a possible effect on calcium influx. Coronary artery relaxation was examined in ovariectomized dogs treated with oestrogen, progesterone, or oestrogen plus progesterone therapy.[170] While progesterone alone minimally affected endothelium-dependent responses, the relaxation response to ACh was less in the combined oestrogen plus progesterone group than the oestrogen alone group. The authors concluded that progesterone antagonizes the stimulatory effect of oestrogen on the production of NO. In a study in surgically postmenopausal cynomolgus monkeys with diet-induced atherosclerosis, Williams and colleagues investigated the effect of added cyclic or continuous medroxyprogesterone acetate (MPA) to conjugated equine oestrogen treatment on coronary vasoreactivity.[171] Whilst oestrogen alone augmented endothelium-dependent dilatation to ACh, the addition of either cyclic or continuous MPA to the oestrogen decreased the ACh-induced dilatation (Figure 8). This suggests that the type of progestogen used in hormone therapy may determine the effects on vascular reactivity. A recent study investigated the effect of oral

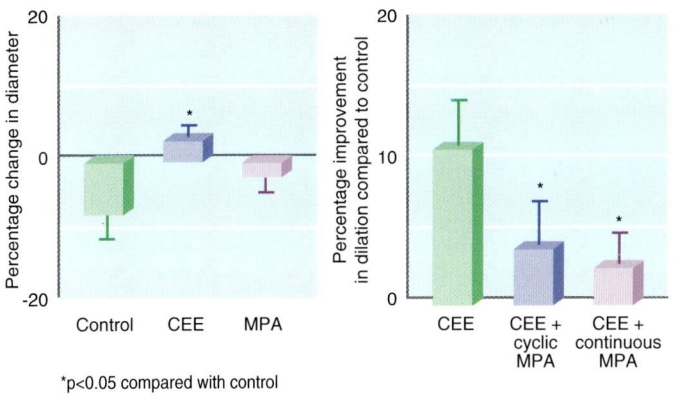

*p<0.05 compared with control

Figure 8.
*The addition of medroxyprogesterone acetate (MPA) reduces oestrogen-induced coronary dilatation to ACh in ovariectomized animals. CEE = conjugated equine oestrogen. (JACC 1994; **24**: 1757–1761).*

MPA versus intravaginal progesterone combined with oral 17β-oestradiol on exercise-induced myocardial ischaemia in post-menopausal women with proven coronary artery disease. Preliminary findings demonstrate a reversal of the beneficial effect of oestrogen therapy with oral MPA, but not intravaginal progesterone, on time to 1 mm ST-segment depression (a sign of myocardial ischaemia).[172] These findings suggest that the progestogen used in association with oestrogen must be carefully chosen when postmenopausal women with coronary heart disease are prescribed hormone therapy.

The evidence of the vascular effects of progestogens to date does not support the administration of progesterone alone for cardiovascular protection or treatment. Recent evidence does suggest that there is little foundation for the worries about the addition of a progestogen to oestrogen therapy with regard to cardiovascular disease risk.

Vascular effects of phyto-oestrogens

Flavanoids are secondary metabolites which occur naturally in all plant families.[173,174] The flavanoids occur in several structurally and biosynthetically related classes; the isoflavones, flavones and chalones are characteristic of a more limited number of plant families. The isoflavones genistein, daidzein and formononetin have previously been reported to be weak oestrogens.[175–177] There are structural similarities between the steroidal nucleus of 17β-oestradiol and the rigid ring structure of the flavanoids. It has subsequently been demonstrated that several flavones (7,8-benzoflavone, chrysin and apigenin) act as inhibitors of the aromatase cytochrome P-450.[178] This enzyme is responsible for synthesizing oestrogens from androgenic precursors and these flavones exert their inhibition by competing with substrate for binding to the catalytic site of the enzyme. Recently it was shown that hydroxylated flavanoids — including chalones (isoliquiritigenin, phloretin), isoflavones (genistein), flavones (agipenin) and flavonones — interact directly with the oestrogen receptor.[179]

Genistein is a tyrosine kinase inhibitor.[180] It blocks L-type calcium currents in vascular smooth muscle cells[181] and potently and reversibly blocks potassium current in pulmonary artery cells.[182]

In vitro studies indicate that genistein has effects on the coagulation system. Genistein prevents thromboxane A_2 and collagen-induced platelet activation.[183] Genistein-induced tyrosine kinase inhibition prevents thrombin-induced platelet activation[184,185] and aggregation.[186] Endothelial cell proliferation and *in vitro* angiogenesis has been shown to be inhibited by genistein.[187]

It has recently been discovered that the isoflavone, genistein, can inhibit ACh-induced coronary vasoconstriction in atherosclerotic cynomolgus monkeys in a very similar way to oestrogen.[188] Female monkeys with diet-induced atherosclerosis were fed diets containing soy protein with or without phyto-oestrogens for six months. Quantitative coronary angiography was performed in all animals at the end of the treatment period, and animals receiving phyto-oestrogens also underwent a 20-minute intravenous infusion of genistein. Both long-term treatment with phyto-oestrogens and short-term genistein administration enhanced the dilator response to ACh.

Lipids

Dietary soy proteins are known to lower cholesterol and a recent study has demonstrated a beneficial effect of genistein on lipid profile in cynomolgus monkeys fed soy protein with or without the addition of genistein.[189] A meta-analysis of studies which investigated the relationship between soy protein consumption and serum lipid concentration found a 9.3 per cent decrease in total cholesterol, a 12.9 per cent decrease in LDL-C and a non-significant 2.4 per cent increase in HDL-C in subjects consuming an average of 47 g of soy protein per day.[190]

Relevance of vascular effects of phyto-oestrogens to CVD prevention and therapy

As well as evidence that ovarian oestrogens have cardiovascular protective effects there is evidence that dietary oestrogens may also confer some cardiovascular protection. Epidemiological data suggest a reduction in incidence of coronary heart disease in humans who have a high intake of phyto-oestrogens,[191] and high levels of the phyto-oestrogen genistein are suggested as an explanation for the infrequency of hot flushes and menopausal symptoms in Japanese women.[192] The effect of flavanoid intake on myocardial infarction and mortality has been studied in elderly men (aged 65–84 years), followed up for five years. Flavanoid intake was inversely associated with incidence of myocardial infarction and mortality (a non-significant trend), suggesting that regularly consumed flavanoids may reduce the risk of death from CHD in elderly men.[193] A cross-sectional correlation study to determine whether flavanoid intake explains differences in mortality rates from chronic diseases between populations demonstrated that dietary flavanoids explained 25 per cent of total CHD mortality variance across the cohorts. Smoking, saturated fat and flavanoid consumption together accounted for 90 per cent of the variance.[194]

These epidemiological data may possibly be explained by the emerging data on the vascular effects of phyto-oestrogens (genistein in particular) on vascular reactivity and risk factors for cardiovascular disease. If these preliminary data can be reproduced in humans then phyto-oestrogens may represent another therapeutic option in menopausal women with coronary heart disease, and a novel therapeutic option for men with coronary heart disease: an oestrogen without reproductive effects.

Vascular effects of testosterone

The fact that premenopausal women have a lower incidence of coronary heart disease and myocardial infarction than men of a similar age has led to the notion that testosterone may predispose to coronary artery disease. However, there has been no direct evidence linking testosterone administration to an increased incidence of coronary heart disease and myocardial infarction. Indeed, testosterone has been shown to have beneficial effects on risk factors for coronary heart disease as well as on vascular reactivity.

Phillips et al,[195] in a study examining the effect of risk factors (including oestradiol and testosterone) on predicting myocardial infarction in males who had not had a previous myocardial infarction, raised the possibility that hypotestosteronaemia in men may be a risk factor for coronary atherosclerosis. This study and others[196–198] demonstrated a positive correlation between testosterone and high-density lipoprotein cholesterol (HDL-C), suggesting that testosterone may be cardioprotective through a beneficial effect on lipoproteins. Others have reported that high doses of testosterone can have a negative effect on HDL-C levels,[199] suggesting a dose-dependent effect.

The effects of experimentally induced hyperandrogenism have been studied in atherosclerotic female cynomolgus monkeys.[200] Animals treated with androgens (androstenedione and oestrone, or testosterone) demonstrated exacerbation of atherosclerosis compared to untreated controls. The atherogenic effects of testosterone were independent of plasma lipoproteins. Interestingly, however, hyperandrogenism reversed atherosclerosis-related impairment of endothelium-dependent vasodilator responses. The relevance of these data, in female animals given normal male levels of androgens, to the human male is unknown. Although the atherosclerotic process was more advanced in the testosterone-treated animals, these animals demonstrated ACh-induced coronary artery dilatation compared to a null or constrictor response in control animals. This suggests that any adverse effect of testosterone on CHD is not due to abnormalities in coronary vasomotion, but may involve effects on atheroma formation and progression.

Testosterone is negatively associated with the haemostatic risk factors plasminogen activator inhibitor-1 (PAI-1),[201,202] factor VII[203,204] and fibrinogen,[195] suggesting that low testosterone levels may be a risk factor for thrombogenesis. Intramuscular injections of testosterone cypionate increase thromboxane A2 receptor density in human platelets and aggregation response, however.[205]

The effect of testosterone on the coronary circulation in humans is unknown; however, recent data show testosterone-induced relaxation in precontracted rabbit coronary arteries and aorta, with or without endothelium (Figure 9).[206] Similar results were obtained from male and non-pregnant female rabbits. The relaxing response of testosterone in the coronary artery was significantly greater than in the aorta. There were significant differences in the relaxing response to testosterone compared to testosterone analogues. Testosterone was the most potent relaxing agent, suggesting that there may be a structure-function relationship in the relaxing response. A recent *in vivo* study in dogs investigated the effect of intracoronary testosterone in coronary conductance and resistance arteries.[207] Increasing doses of testosterone significantly

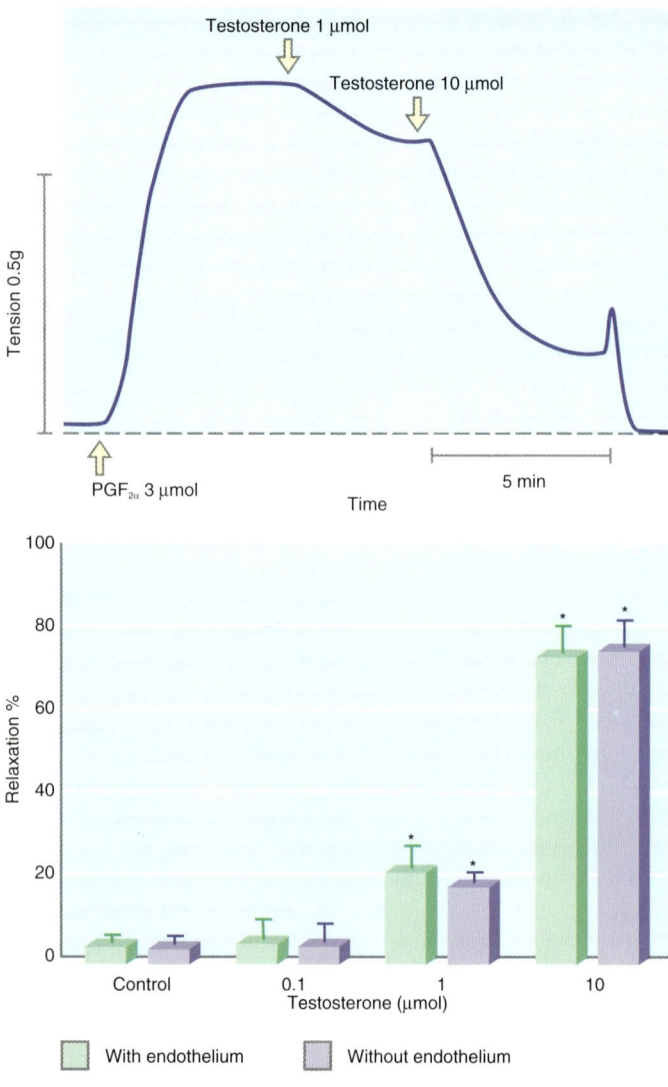

Figure 9.
*Trace and percentage relaxation to testosterone of coronary artery rings precontracted with PGF$_{2\alpha}$. (Circulation 1995; **91**: 1154–1160).*

* Significant differences in comparison with control, p<0.01

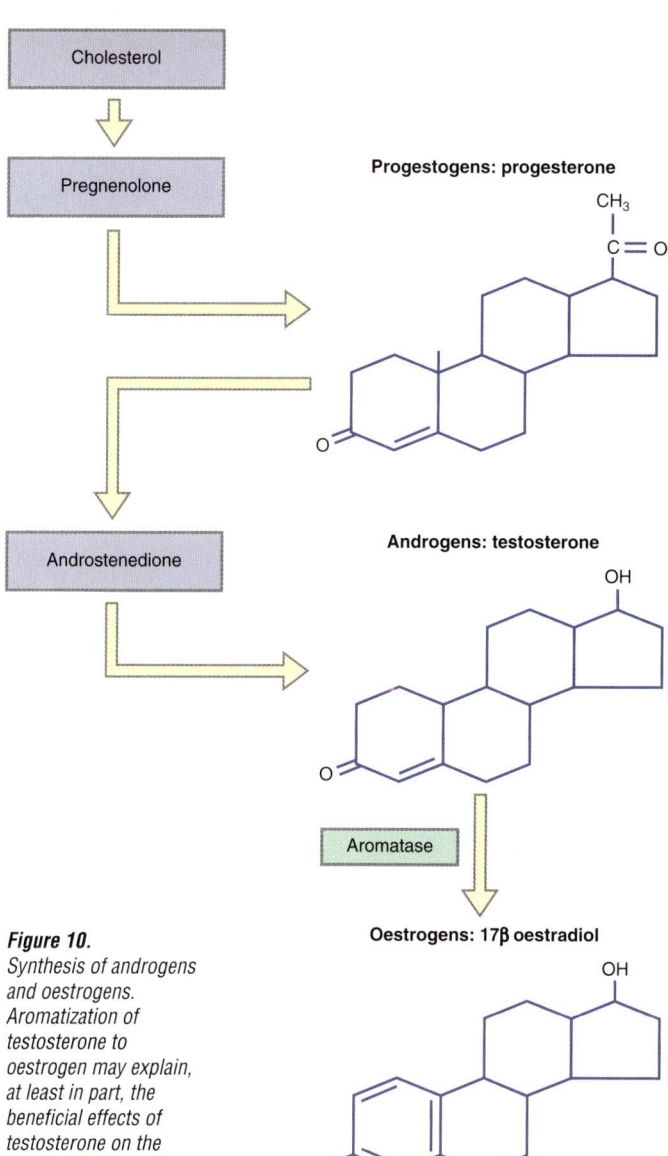

Progestogens: progesterone

Androgens: testosterone

Aromatase

Oestrogens: 17β oestradiol

Figure 10.
Synthesis of androgens and oestrogens. Aromatization of testosterone to oestrogen may explain, at least in part, the beneficial effects of testosterone on the cardiovascular system.

45

increased coronary diameter and blood flow in both male and female animals. Experiments using the inhibitor of NO synthesis, N^{ω}-nitro-L-arginine methyl ester, resulted in a non-significant attenuation of this response. Antagonism of ATP-sensitive potassium channels by glibenclamide attenuated testosterone-induced dilatation in resistance but not epicardial arteries. Testosterone is aromatized to oestradiol (Figure 10), raising the possibility that oestradiol accounts for the vascular effects attributed to testosterone. However, inhibition of the classic oestrogen receptor did not affect testosterone-induced vasodilatation.

These data demonstrate that testosterone can influence the regulation of coronary tone, and this may be one of the explanations as to why testosterone has previously been shown to have beneficial effects on anginal symptoms and on parameters of myocardial ischaemia in patients treated with this hormone.[208–212]

Relevance of vascular effects
of testosterone to CVD prevention
and treatment

Myocardial ischaemia

Testosterone therapy in men has been shown to have a beneficial effect on angina pectoris[208–211] and on exercise-induced ST segment depression in patients with angina pectoris.[212] A double blind study was carried out in 50 men who had ST segment depression after exercise.[212] It was shown that after four to eight weeks' treatment with testosterone or placebo there was a significant decrease in the exercise-induced extent of ST segment depression by testosterone when compared to placebo. The mechanisms by which testosterone decreased post-exercise ST segment depression were not established, but the recent evidence suggesting that testosterone may have relaxing effects on the coronary arteries suggests that the mechanism may involve an increase in blood supply to the myocardium.

References

1. Eaker E, Chesebro JH, Sacks FM, Wenger NK, Whisnant JP, Winston M. Cardiovascular disease in women. *Circulation* 1993; **88**: 1999–2009.

2. Pinsky JL, Jette AM, Branch LG, Kannel WB, Feinleib M. The Framingham Disability Study: relationship of various coronary heart disease manifestations to disability in older persons living in the community. *Am J Public Health* 1990; **80**: 1363–1367.

3. Steingart RM, Packer M, Hamm P, et al. Sex differences in the management of coronary artery disease. Survival and Ventricular Enlargement Investigators. *N Engl J Med* 1991; **325**: 226–230.

4. Ayanian JZ, Epstein AM. Differences in the use of procedures between men and women hospitalised for coronary heart disease. *N Engl J Med* 1991; **325**: 221–225.

5. Petticrew M, McKee M, Jones J. Coronary artery surgery: are women discriminated against? *Br Med J* 1993; **306**: 1164–1166.

6. Mark DB, Shaw LK, DeLong ER, Califf RM, Pryor DB. Absence of sex bias in the referral of patients for cardiac catheterization. *Circulation* 1994; **330**: 1101–1106.

7. Gomez-Marin O, Folsom AR, Kottke TE, et al. Improvement in long-term survival among patients hospitalized with acute myocardial infarction. *N Engl J Med* 1987; **316**: 1353–1359.

8. Dittrich H, Gilpin E, Nicod P, Cali G, Henning H, Ross J, Jr. Acute myocardial infarction in women: influence of gender on mortality and prognostic variables. *Am J Cardiol* 1988; **62**: 1–7.

9. Puletti M, Sunseri L, Curione M, Erba SM, Borgia C. Acute myocardial infarction: sex related differences in prognosis. *Am Heart J* 1984; **108**: 63–66.

10. White HD, Barbash GI, Modan M, et al. After correcting for worse baseline characteristics, women treated with thrombolytic therapy for acute myocardial infarction have the same mortality and morbidity as men except for a higher incidence of hemorrhagic stroke. *Circulation* 1993; **88**: 2097–2103.

11. Kelsey SF, James M, Holubkov AL, Holubkov R, Cowley MJ, Detre KM. Results of percutaneous transluminal coronary angioplasty in women. *Circulation* 1993; **87** No 3: 720–727.

12. O'Connor GT, Morton JR, Diehl MJ, et al. Differences between men and women in hospital mortality associated with coronary artery bypass graft surgery. *Circulation* 1993; **88**: 2104–2110.

13. Colditz GA, Willett WC, Stampfer MJ, Rosner B, Speizer FE, Hennekens CH. Menopause and the risk of coronary heart disease in women. *N Engl J Med* 1987; **316**: 1105–1110.

14. Stampfer MJ, Colditz GA. Estrogen replacement therapy and coronary heart disease: a quantitative assessment of the epidemiologic evidence. *Prev Med* 1991; **20**: 47–63.

15. Pfeffer RI, Kurosaki TT, Charlton SK. Estrogen use and blood pressure in later life. *Am J Epidemiol* 1979; **110**: 469–478.

16. Hammond CB, Jelovsek FR, Lee KL, Creasman WT, Parker RT. Effects of long-term estrogen replacement therapy. I. Metabolic effects. *Am J Obstet Gynecol* 1979; **133**: 525–536.

17. Hazzard WR. Estrogen replacement and cardiovascular disease: serum lipids and blood pressure effects. *Am J Obstet Gynecol* 1989; **161**: 1847–1853.

18. Luotola H. Blood pressure and hemodynamics in postmenopausal women during estradiol-17 beta substitution. *Ann Clin Res* 1983; **15** (Suppl 38): 1–121.

19. The Postmenopausal Estrogen/Progestin Interventions Trial Writing Group. Effects of estrogen or estrogen/progestin regimens on heart disease risk factors in postmenopausal women. *JAMA* 1995; **273**: 199–208.

20. Lip GY, Beevers M, Churchill D, Beevers DG. Hormone replacement therapy and blood pressure in hypertensive women. *J Hum Hypertens* 1994; **8**: 491–494.

21. Henderson BE, Paginini-Hill A, Rossk RK. Decreased mortality in users of estrogen replacement therapy. *Arch Intern Med* 1991; **151**: 75–78.

22. Stampfer MJ, Willett WC, Colditz GA, Rosner B, Speizer FE, Hennekens CH. A prospective study of postmenopausal estrogen therapy and coronary heart disease. *N Engl J Med* 1985; **313**: 1044–1049.

23. Adam S, Williams V, Vessey MP. Cardiovascular disease and hormone replacement treatment: a pilot case-control study. *Br Med J* 1981; **282**: 1277–1278.

24. Paganini-Hill A, Ross RK, Henderson BE. Postmenopausal oestrogen treatment and stroke: a prospective study. *Br Med J* 1988; **297**: 519–522.

25. Falkeborn M, Persson I, Terent A, Adami HO, Lithell H, Bergstrom R. Hormone replacement therapy and the risk of stroke. Follow-up of a population-based cohort in Sweden. *Arch Intern Med* 1993; **153**: 1201–1209.

26. Byrd BF, Jr., Burch JC, Vaughn WK. The impact of long term estrogen support after hysterectomy. A report of 1016 cases. *Ann Surg* 1977; **185**: 574–580.

27. Hunt K, Vessey M, McPherson K. Mortality in a cohort of long-term users of hormone replacement therapy: an updated analysis. *Br J Obstet Gynaecol* 1990; **97**: 1080–1086.

28. Wilson PW, Garrison RJ, Castelli WP. Postmenopausal estrogen use, cigarette smoking, and cardiovascular morbidity in women over 50. The Framingham Study. *N Engl J Med* 1985; **313**: 1038–1043.

29. Bush TL, Barrett-Connor E, Cowan LD, et al. Cardiovascular mortality and noncontraceptive use of estrogen in women: results from the Lipid Research Clinics Program Follow-up Study. *Circulation* 1987; **75**: 1102–1109.

30. Petitti DB, Perlman JA, Sidney S. Noncontraceptive estrogens and mortality: long-term follow-up of women in the Walnut Creek Study. *Obstet Gynecol* 1987; **70**: 289–293.

31. Finucane FF, Madans JH, Bush TL, Wolf PH, Kleinman JC. Decreased risk of stroke among postmenopausal hormone users. Results from a national cohort. *Arch Intern Med* 1993; **153**: 73–79.

32. Grady D, Rubin SM, Petitti DB, et al. Cummings SR. Hormone therapy to prevent disease and prolong life in postmenopausal women. *Ann Intern Med* 1992; **117**: 1016–1037.

33. Stevenson JC, Crook D, Godsland IF. Influence of age and menopause on serum lipids and lipoproteins in healthy women. *Atherosclerosis* 1993; **98**: 83–90.

34. Godsland IF, Wynn V, Crook D, Miller NE. Sex, plasma lipoproteins, and atherosclerosis: prevailing assumptions and outstanding questions. *Am Heart J* 1987; **114**: 1467–1503.

35. Nabulsi AA, Folsom AR, White A, Patsch W, Heiss G, Wu KK, Szklo M. Association of hormone-replacement therapy with various cardiovascular risk factors in postmenopausal women. The Atherosclerosis Risk in Communities Study Investigators. *N Engl J Med* 1993; **328**: 1069–1075.

36. Soma M, Fumagalli R, Paoletti R, et al. Plasma Lp(a) concentration after oestrogen and progestagen in postmenopausal women. *Lancet* 1991; **337**: 612.

37. Walsh BW, Schiff I, Rosner B, Greenberg L, Ravnikar V, Sacks FM. Effects of postmenopausal estrogen replacement on the concentrations and metabolism of plasma lipoproteins. *N Engl J Med* 1991; **325**: 1196–1204.

38. Barrett-Connor E, Wingard DL, Criqui MH. Postmenopausal estrogen use and heart disease risk factors in the 1980s. Rancho Bernardo, Calif, revisited. *JAMA* 1989; **261**: 2095–2100.

39. Lobo RA. Clinical review 27: effects of hormonal replacement on lipids and lipoproteins in postmenopausal women. *J Clin Endocrinol Metab* 1991; **73**: 925–930.

40. Abbott WG, Lillioja S, Young AA, et al. Relationships between plasma lipoprotein concentrations and insulin action in an obese hyperinsulinemic population. *Diabetes* 1987; **36**: 897–904.

41. Stevenson JC, Crook D, Godsland IF, Collins P, Whitehead MI. Hormone replacement therapy and the cardiovascular system nonlipid effects. *Drugs* 1994; **47** (Suppl 2): 35–41.

42. Godsland IF, Gangar KF, Walton C, et al. Insulin resistance, secretion, and elimination in postmenopausal women receiving oral or transdermal hormone replacement therapy. *Metabolism* 1993; **42**: 846–853.

43. Ley CJ, Lees B, Stevenson JC. Sex- and menopause-associated changes in body-fat distribution. *Am J Clin Nutr* 1992; **55**: 950–954.

44. Haarbo J, Marslew U, Gotfredsen A, Christiansen C. Postmenopausal hormone replacement therapy prevents central distribution of body fat after menopause. *Metabolism* 1991; **40**: 1323–1326.

45. Daly E, Vessey MP, Hawkins MM, Carson JL, Gough P, Marsh S. Risk of venous thromboembolism in users of hormone replacement therapy. *Lancet* 1996; **348**: 977–980.

46. Jick H, Derby LE, Wald-Meyers M, Vasilakis C, Newton KM. Risk of hospital admission for idiopathic venous thromboembolism among users of postmenopausal oestrogens. *Lancet* 1996; **348**: 981–983.

47. Grodstein F, Stampfer MJ, Goldhaber SZ, et al. Prospective study of exogenous hormones and risk of pulmonary embolism in women. *Lancet* 1996; **348**: 983–987.

48. Scarabin PY, Bonithon-Kopp C, Bara L, Malmejac A, Guize L, Samama M. Factor VII activation and menopausal status. *Thromb Res* 1990; **57**: 227–234.

49. Folsom AR, Wu KK, Davis CE, Conlan MG, Sorlie PD, Szklo M. Population correlates of plasma fibrinogen and factor VII, putative cardiovascular risk factors. *Atherosclerosis* 1991; **91**: 191–205.

50. Heinrich J, Sandkamp M, Kokott R, Schulte H, Assmann G. Relationship of lipoprotein(a) to variables of coagulation and fibrinolysis in a healthy population. *Clin Chem* 1991; **37**: 1950–1954.

51. Gebara OCE, Mittleman MA, Sutherland P, et al. Association between increased estrogen status and increased fibrinolytic potential in the Framingham Offspring study. *Circulation* 1995; **91**: 1952–1958.

52. Devor M, Barrett-Connor E, Renvall M, Feigal D, Jr., Ramsdell J. Estrogen replacement therapy and the risk of venous thrombosis. *Am J Med* 1992; **92**: 275–282.

53. Lowe GDO, Greer IA, Cooke TG. Risk of and prophylaxis for venous thromboembolism in hospital patients. Thromboembolic Risk Factors (THRIFT) Consensus Group. *Br Med J* 1992; **305**: 567–574.

54. Sudhir K, Chou TM, Mullen WL, et al. Mechanisms of estrogen-induced vasodilation: in vivo studies in canine coronary conductance and resistance arteries. *J Am Coll Cardiol* 1995; **26**: 807–814.

55. Williams JK, Adams MR, Klopfenstein HS. Estrogen modulates responses of atherosclerotic coronary arteries. *Circulation* 1990; **81**: 1680–1687.

56. Williams JK, Adams MR, Herrington DM, Clarkson TB. Short-term administration of estrogen and vascular responses of atherosclerotic coronary arteries. *J Am Coll Cardiol* 1992; **20**: 452–457.

57. Reis SE, Gloth ST, Blumenthal RS, et al. Ethinyl estradiol acutely attenuates abnormal coronary vasomotor responses to acetylcholine in postmenopausal women. *Circulation* 1994; **89**: 52–60.

58. Gilligan DM, Quyyumi AA, Cannon RO, III. Effects of physiological levels of estrogen on coronary vasomotor function in postmenopausal women. *Circulation* 1994; **89**: 2545–2551.

59. Collins P, Rosano GMC, Sarrel PM, et al. Estradiol-17β attenuates acetylcholine-induced coronary arterial constriction in women but not men with coronary heart disease. *Circulation* 1995; **92**: 24–30.

60. Herrington DM, Braden GA, Williams JK, Morgan TM. Endothelial-dependent coronary vasomotor responsiveness in postmenopausal women with and without estrogen replacement therapy. *Am J Cardiol* 1994; **73**: 951–952.

61. Magness RR, Rosenfeld CR. Local and systemic estradiol-17 beta: effects on uterine and systemic vasodilation. *Am J Physiol* 1989; **256**: E536–E542.

62. Volterrani M, Rosano GMC, Coats A, Beale C, Collins P. Estrogen acutely increases peripheral blood flow in post-menopausal women. *Am J Med* 1995; **99**: 119–122.

63. Riedel M, Oeltermann A, Mugge A, Creutzig A, Rafflenbeul W, Lichtlen P. Vascular responses to 17 beta-oestradiol in postmenopausal women. *Eur J Clin Invest* 1995; **25**: 44–47.

64. Hashimoto M, Akishita M, Eto M, et al. Modulation of endothelium-dependent flow-mediated dilatation of the brachial artery by sex and menstrual cycle. *Circulation* 1995; **92**: 3431–3435.

65. Gilligan DM, Badar DM, Panza JA, Quyyumi AA, Cannon RO, III. Acute vascular effects of estrogen in post-menopausal women. *Circulation* 1994; **90**: 786–791.

66. Lieberman EH, Gerhard MD, Uehata A, et al. Estrogen improves endothelium-dependent, flow-mediated vasodila-tion in postmenopausal women. *Ann Intern Med* 1994; **121**: 936–941.

67. Ganger KF, Vyas S, Whitehead M, Crook D, Meire H, Campbell S. Pulsatility index in internal carotid artery in rela-tion to transdermal oestradiol and time since menopause. *Lancet* 1991; **338**: 839–842.

68. McGill HC, Jr.. Sex steroid hormone receptors in the cardio-vascular system. *Postgrad Med* 1989; 64–68.

69. Kahn D, Zeng Q, Kajani M, et al. The effect of different types of hepatic injury on the estrogen and androgen receptor activity of liver. *J Invest Surg* 1989; **2**: 125–133.

70. Losordo DW, Kearney M, Kim EA, Jekanowski J, Isner JM. Variable expression of the estrogen receptor in normal and atherosclerotic coronary arteries of premenopausal women. *Circulation* 1994; **89**: 1501–1510.

71. Collins P, Sheppard M, Beale CM, Dowsett M. The classical estrogen receptor is not found in human coronary arteries. *Circulation* 1995; **92**: I–37.(abstract).

72. Venkov CD, Rankin AB, Vaughan DE. Identification of authentic estrgoen receptor in cultured endothelial cells. A potential mechanism for steroid hormone regulation of endothelial function. *Circulation* 1996; **94**: 727–733.

73. Kim-Schulze S, McGowan KA, Hubchak SC, et al. Expression of an estrogen receptor by human coronary artery and umbilical vein endothelial cells. *Circulation* 1996; **94**: 1402–1407.

74. Kuiper GG, Enmark E, Pelto-Huikko M, Nilsson S, Gustafsson JA. Cloning of a novel receptor expressed in rat prostate and ovary. *Proc Natl Acad Sci USA* 1996; **93**: 5925–5930.

75. Williams SP, Shackelford DP, Iams SG, Mustafa SJ. Endothelium-dependent relaxation in estrogen-treated spontaneously hypertensive rats. *Eur J Pharmacol* 1988; **145**: 205–207.

76. Gisclard V, Miller VM, Vanhoutte PM. Effect of 17β-estradiol on endothelium-dependent responses in the rabbit. *J Pharmacol Exp Ther* 1988; **244**: 19–22.

77. Weiner CP, Lizasoain I, Baylis SA, Knowles RG, Charles IG, Moncada S. Induction of calcium-dependent nitric oxide synthases by sex hormones. *Proc Natl Acad Sci USA* 1994; **91**: 5212–5216.

78. Dubey RK, Overbeck HW. Culture of rat mesenteric arteriolar smooth muscle cells: effects of platelet-derived growth factor, angiotensin, and nitric oxide on growth. *Cell Tissue Res* 1994; **275**: 133–141.

79. Sack MN, Rader DJ, Cannon RO, III. Oestrogen and inhibition of oxidation of low-density lipoproteins in postmenopausal women. *Lancet* 1994; **343**: 269–270.

80. Simon BC, Cunningham LD, Cohen RA. Oxidized low density lipoproteins cause contraction and inhibit endothelium-dependent relaxation in the pig coronary artery. *J Clin Invest* 1990; **86**: 75–79.

81. Hayashi T, Fukuto JM, Ignarro LJ, Chaudhuri G. Basal release of nitric oxide from aortic rings is greater in female rabbits than in male rabbits: implications for atherosclerosis. *Proc Natl Acad Sci USA* 1992; **89**: 11259–11263.

82. Collins P, Shay J, Jiang C, Moss J. Nitric oxide accounts for dose-dependent estrogen-mediated coronary relaxation following acute estrogen withdrawal. *Circulation* 1994; **90**: 1964–1968.

83. Futo J, Shay J, Holt J, Moss J. Estrogen and progesterone withdrawal increases cerebral vasoreactivity to serotonin in rabbit basilar artery. *Life Sci* 1992; **50**: 1165–1172.

84. Shay J, Badrov N, Attele A, Levinson M, Moss J. Estrogen antagonises endothelin-1 vasoconstriction in rabbit basilar artery. *Anesth Analg* 1993; A561.

85. Kharitonov SA, Logan-Sinclair RB, Busset CM, Shinebourne EA. Peak expiratory nitric oxide differences in men and women: relation to the menstrual cycle. *Br Heart J* 1994; **72**: 243–245.

86. Schray-Utz B, Zeiher AM, Busse R. Expression of constitutive NO synthase in cultured endothelial cells is enhanced by 17β-estradiol. *Circulation* 1993; **88**: 1–80 (abstract).

87. Caulin-Glaser TL, Sessa W, Sarrel P, Bender J. The effect of 17β-estradiol on human endothelial cell nitric oxide production. *Circulation* 1994; **90**: I–30 (abstract).

88. Gorodeski GI, Yang T, Levy MN, Goldfarb J, Utian WH. Effects of estrogen in vivo on coronary vascular resistance in perfused rabbit hearts. *Am J Physiol* 1995; **269**: R1333–R1338.

89. Van Buren G, Yang D, Clark KE. Estrogen-induced uterine vasodilatation is antagonized by L-nitroarginine methyl ester, an inhibitor of nitric oxide synthesis. *Am J Obstet Gynecol* 1992; **16**: 828–833.

90. Hishikawa K, Nakaki T, Marumo T, Suzuki H, Kato R, Saruta T. Up-regulation of nitric oxide synthase by estradiol in human aortic endothelial cells. *FEBS Lett* 1995; **360**: 291–293.

91. Goetz RM, Morano I, Calovini T, Studer R, Holtz J. Increased expression of endothelial constitutive nitric oxide synthase in rat aorta during pregnancy. *Biochem Biophys Res Commun* 1994; **205**: 905–910.

92. Jiang C, Sarrel PM, Lindsay DC, Poole-Wilson PA, Collins P. Endothelium-independent relaxation of rabbit coronary artery by 17β-estradiol in vitro. *Br J Pharmacol* 1991; **104**: 1033–1037.

93. Chester AH, Jiang C, Borland JA, Yacoub MH, Collins P. Estrogen relaxes human epicardial coronary arteries through non-endothelium-dependent mechanisms. *Cor Art Dis* 1995; **6**: 417–422.

94. Stice SL, Ford SP, Rosazza JP, Van-Orden DE. Interaction of 4-hydroxylated estradiol and potential-sensitive Ca^{2+} channels in altering uterine blood flow during the estrous cycle and early pregnancy in gilts. *Biol Reprod* 1987; **36**: 369–375.

95. Jiang C, Poole-Wilson PA, Sarrel PM, Mochizuki S, Collins P, MacLeod KT. Effect of 17β-estradiol on contraction, Ca^{2+} current and intracellular free Ca^{2+} in guinea-pig isolated cardiac myocytes. *Br J Pharmacol* 1992; **106**: 739–745.

96. Han SZ, Karaki H, Ouchi Y, Akishita M, Orimo H. 17β-estradiol inhibits Ca^{2+} influx and Ca^{2+} release induced by thromboxane A2 in porcine coronary artery. *Circulation* 1995; **91**: 2619–2626.

97. Zhang F, Ram JL, Standley PR, Sowers JR. 17β-estradiol attenuates voltage-dependent Ca^{2+} currents in A7r5 vascular smooth muscle cell line. *Am J Physiol* 1994; **266**: C975–C980.

98. Hardy SP, Valverde MA. Novel plasma membrane action of estrogen and antiestrogens revealed by their regulation of a large conductance chloride channel. *FASEB J* 1994; **8**: 760–765.

99. Lloyd T, Weisz J. Direct inhibition of tyrosine hydroxylase activity by catechol estrogens. *J Biol Chem* 1978; **253**: 4841–4843.

100. Kvetnansky R, Fukuhara K, Pacak K, Cizza G, Goldstein DS, Kopin IJ. Endogenous glucocorticoids restrain catecholamine synthesis and release at rest and during immobilization stress in rats. *Endocrinology* 1993; **133**: 1411–1419.

101. Lindheim SR, Legro RS, Bernstein L, et al. Behavioral stress responses in premenopausal and postmenopausal women and the effects of estrogen. *Am J Obstet Gynecol* 1992; **167**: 1831–1836.

102. Cruickshank JM, Smith JC. The beta-receptor, atheroma and cardiovascular damage. *Pharmacol Ther* 1989; **42**: 385–404.

103. McEwen BS, Parsons B. Gonadal steroid action on the brain: neurochemistry and neuropharmacology. *Annu Rev Pharmacol Toxicol* 1982; **22**: 555–598.

104. Luine VN. Estradiol increases choline acetyltransferase activity in specific basal forebrain nuclei and projection areas of female rats. *Exp Neurol* 1985; **89**: 484–490.

105. O'Malley CA, Hautamaki RD, Kelley M, Meyer EM. Effects of ovariectomy and estradiol benzoate on high affinity choline uptake, ACh synthesis, and release from rat cerebral cortical synaptosomes. *Brain Res* 1987; **403**: 389–392.

106. Ryne SM, Goldberger AL, Pincus SM, Mietus J, Lipsitz LA. Gender- and age-related differences in heart rate dynamics: Are women more complex than men? *J Am Coll Cardiol* 1994; **24**: 1700–1707.

107. Oliver JA, Sciacca RR. Local generation of angiotensin II as a mechanism of regulation of peripheral vascular tone in the rat. *J Clin Invest* 1984; **74**: 1247–1251.

108. Nakamaru M, Jackson EK, Inagami T. Beta-adrenoceptor-mediated release of angiotensin II from mesenteric arteries. *Am J Physiol* 1986; **250**: H144–H148.

109. Jackson TR, Blair LA, Marshall J, Goedert M, Hanley MR. The mas oncogene encodes an angiotensin receptor. *Nature* 1988; **335**: 437–440.

110. Ryan US, Ryan JW, Whitaker C, Chiu A. Localization of angiotensin converting enzyme (kininase II). II. Immunocytochemistry and immunofluorescence. *Tissue Cell* 1976; **8**: 125–145.

111. Okunishi H, Miyazaki M, Okamura T, Toda N. Different distribution of two types of angiotensin II-generating enzymes in the aortic wall. *Biochem Biophys Res Commun* 1987; **149**: 1186–1192.

112. Cheng DY, Gruetter CA. Chronic estrogen alters contractile responsiveness to angiotensin II and norepinephrine in female rat aorta. *Eur J Pharmacol* 1992; **215**: 171–176.

113. Magness RR, Parker CR, Jr., Rosenfeld CR. Systemic and uterine responses to chronic infusion of estradiol-17 beta. *Am J Physiol* 1993; **265**: E690–E698.

114. Proudler AJ, Hasib Ahmed AI, Crook D, Fogelman I, Rymer JM, Stevenson JC. Hormone replacement therapy and serum angiotensin-converting-enzyme activity in post-menopausal women. *Lancet* 1995; **346**: 89–90.

115. Mancini GB, Henry GC, Macaya C, et al. Angiotensin-converting enzyme inhibition with quinapril improves endothelial vasomotor dysfunction in patients with coronary artery disease. The TREND (Trial on Reversing ENdothelial Dysfunction) study. *Circulation* 1996; **94**: 258–265.

116. Wiemer G, Scholkens BA, Becker RH, Busse R. Ramiprilat enhances endothelial autacoid formation by inhibiting breakdown of endothelium-derived bradykinin. *Hypertension* 1991; **18**: 558–563.

117. Jiang C, Sarrel PM, Poole-Wilson PA, Collins P. Acute effect of 17β-estradiol on rabbit coronary artery contractile responses to endothelin-1. *Am J Physiol* 1992; **263**: H271–H275.

118. Lerman A, Webster MWI, Chesebro JH, et al. Circulating and tissue endothelin immunoreactivity in hypercholesterolemic pigs. *Circulation* 1993; **88**: 2923–2928.

119. Botting R, Vane JR. The receipt and dispatch of chemical messengers by endothelial cells. In: Schrör K, Sinzinger H (eds.) *Prostaglandins in Clinical Research: Cardiovascular System*, New York: Alan R. Liss, Inc., 1989: 1–11.

120. Mendelsohn ME, Karas RH. Estrogen and the blood vessel wall. *Curr Opin Cardiol* 1994; **9**: 619–626.

121. Chang WC, Nakao J, Orimo H, Murota S. Stimulation of prostacyclin biosynthetic activity by estradiol in rat aortic smooth muscle cells in culture. *Biochim Biophys Acta* 1980; **619**: 107–118.

122. Bath PM, Hassall DG, Gladwin AM, Palmer RM, Martin JF. Nitric oxide and prostacyclin. Divergence of inhibitory effects on monocyte chemotaxis and adhesion to endothelium in vitro. *Arterioscler Thromb* 1991; **11**: 254–260.

123. Meredith IT, Yeung AC, Weidinger FF, et al. Role of impaired endothelium-dependent vasodilation in ischemic manifestations of coronary artery disease. *Circulation* 1993; **87** (Suppl V): 56–66.

124. Ludmer PL, Selwyn AP, Shook TL, et al. Paradoxical vasoconstriction induced by acetylcholine in atherosclerotic coronary arteries. *N Engl J Med* 1986; **315**: 1046–1051.

125. Gimbrone MA, Jr., Cybulsky MI, Kume N, Collins T, Resnick N. Vascular endothelium. An integrator of pathophysiological stimuli in atherogenesis. *Ann NY Acad Sci* 1995; **748**: 122–131.

126. Miller ME, Dores GM, Thorpe SL, Akerley WL. Paradoxical influence of estrogenic hormones on platelet-endothelial cell interactions. *Thromb Res* 1994; **74**: 577–594.

127. Raman BB, Standley PR, Rajkumar V, Ram JL, Sowers JR. Effects of estradiol and progesterone on platelet calcium responses. *Am J Hypertens* 1995; **8**: 197–200.

128. Bar J, Tepper R, Fuchs J, Pardo Y, Goldberger S, Ovadia J. The effect of estrogen replacement therapy on platelet aggregation and adenosine triphosphate release in postmenopausal women. *Obstet Gynecol* 1993; **81**: 261–264.

129. Zeiher AM, Fisslthaler B, Schray-Utz B, Busse R. Nitric oxide modulates the expression of monocyte chemoattractant protein 1 in cultured human endothelial cells. *Circ Res* 1995; **76**: 980–986.

130. Radomski MW, Palmer RMJ, Moncada S. Endogenous nitric oxide inhibits human platelet adhesion to vascular endothelium. *Lancet* 1987; **2**: 1057–1058.

131. Henderson BE, Paganini-Hill A, Ross RK. Estrogen replacement therapy and protection from acute myocardial infarction. *Am J Obstet Gynecol* 1988; **159**: 312–317.

132. Jick H, Dinan B, Rothman KJ. Noncontraceptive estrogens and nonfatal myocardial infarction. *JAMA* 1978; **239**: 1407–1409.

133. Falkeborn M, Persson I, Adami HO, et al. The risk of acute myocardial infarction after oestrogen and oestrogen-progestogen replacement. *Br J Obstet Gynaecol* 1992; **99**: 821–828.

134. Ross RK, Paganini-Hill A, Mack TM, Arthur M, Henderson BE. Menopausal oestrogen therapy and protection from death from ischaemic heart disease. *Lancet* 1981; **1**: 858–860.

135. Gruchow HW, Anderson AJ, Barboriak JJ, Sobocinski KA. Postmenopausal use of estrogen and occlusion of coronary arteries. *Am Heart J* 1988; **115**: 954–963.

136. Sullivan JM, Vander Zwaag R, Lemp GF, et al. Postmenopausal estrogen use and coronary atherosclerosis. *Ann Intern Med* 1988; **108**: 358–363.

137. Lichtlen PR, Hugenholtz PG, Rafflenbeul W, Hecker H, Jost S, Deckers JW. Retardation of angiographic progression of coronary artery disease by nifedipine. *Lancet* 1990; **335**: 1109–1113.

138. Waters D, Lesperance J, Francetich M, et al. A controlled clinical trial to assess the effect of a calcium channel blocker on the progression of coronary atherosclerosis. *Circulation* 1990; **82**: 1940–1953.

139. Collins P, Rosano GMC, Jiang C, Lindsay D, Sarrel PM, Poole-Wilson PA. Hypothesis: Cardiovascular protection by oestrogen — a calcium antagonist effect? *Lancet* 1993; **341**: 1264–1265.

140. Adams MR, Kaplan JR, Manuck SB, et al. Inhibition of coronary artery atherosclerosis by 17-beta estradiol in ovariectomized monkeys. Lack of an effect of added progesterone. *Arteriosclerosis* 1990; **10**: 1051–1057.

141. Clarkson TB, Anthony MS, Klein KP. Effects of estrogen treatment on arterial wall structure and function. *Drugs* 1994; **47** (Suppl 2): 42–51.

142. Harrison DG, Ohara Y. Physiologic consequences of increased vascular oxidant stresses in hypercholesterolemia and atherosclerosis: implications for impaired vasomotion. *Am J Cardiol* 1995; **75**: 75B–81B.

143. Steinberg D. Antioxidants in the prevention of human atherosclerosis. Summary of the proceedings of a National Heart, Lung, and Blood Institute Workshop: September 5–6, 1991, Bethesda, Maryland. *Circulation* 1992; **85**: 2337–2344.

144. Steinberg D, Parthasarathy S, Carew TE, Khoo JC, Witztum JL. Beyond cholesterol: modifications of low density lipoprotein that increase its atherogenicity. *N Engl J Med* 1989; **320**: 915–923.

145. Sugioka K, Shimosegawa Y, Nakano M. Estrogens as natural antioxidants of membrane phospholipid peroxidation. *FEBS Lett* 1987; **210**: 37–39.

146. Fischer-Dzoga K, Wissler RW, Vesselinovitch D. The effect of estradiol on the proliferation of rabbit aortic medial tissue culture cells induced by hyperlipemic serum. *Exp Mol Pathol* 1983; **39**: 355–363.

147. O'Brien JE, Peterson ED, Keeler GP, Berdan LG, Ohman EM, Faxon DP. Impact of estrogen replacement therapy on restenosis following percutaneous coronary interventions. *Circulation* 1995; **92**: I–345 (abstract).

148. Fischer GM, Cherian K, Swain ML. Increased synthesis of aortic collagen and elastin in experimental atherosclerosis. Inhibition by contraceptive steroids. *Atherosclerosis* 1981; **39**: 463–467.

149. Beldekas JC, Smith B, Gerstenfeld LC, Sonenshein GE, Franzblau C. Effects of 17 beta-estradiol on the biosynthesis of collagen in cultured bovine aortic smooth muscle cells. *Biochemistry* 1981; **20**: 2162–2167.

150. Fischer GM, Swain ML. Effects of estradiol and progesterone on the increased synthesis of collagen in atherosclerotic rabbit aortas. *Atherosclerosis* 1985; **54**: 177–185.

151. Morales DE, McGowan KA, Grant DS, et al. Estrogen promotes angiogenic activity in human umbilical vein endothelial cells in vitro and in a murine model. *Circulation* 1995; **91**: 755–763.

152. Rosano GMC, Sarrel PM, Poole-Wilson PA, Collins P. Beneficial effect of oestrogen on exercise-induced myocardial ischaemia in women with coronary artery disease. *Lancet* 1993; **342**: 133–136.

153. Panza JA, Quyyumi AA, Brush JE, Epstein SE. Abnormal endothelium-dependent vascular relaxation in patients with essential hypertension. *N Engl J Med* 1990; **323**: 22–27.

154. Likoff W, Segal BL, Kasparian H. Paradox of normal selective coronary arteriograms in patients considered to have unmistakable coronary heart disease. *N Engl J Med* 1967; **276**: 1063–1066.

155. Kemp HG, Jr., Vokonas PS, Cohn PF, Gorlin R. The anginal syndrome associated with normal coronary arteriograms. Report of a six year experience. *Am J Med* 1973; **54**: 735–742.

156. Maseri A, Crea F, Kaski JC, Crake T. Mechanisms of angina pectoris in syndrome X. *J Am Coll Cardiol* 1991; **17**: 499–506.

157. Cannon RO, Epstein SE. 'Microvascular angina' as a cause of chest pain with angiographically normal coronary arteries. *Am J Cardiol* 1988; **61**: 1338–1343.

158. Rosano GMC, Lindsay DC, Poole-Wilson PA. Syndrome X: an hypothesis for cardiac pain without ischaemia. *Cardiologia* 1991; **36**: 885–895.

159. Opherk D, Zebe H, Weihe E, et al. Reduced coronary dilatory capacity and ultrastructural changes of the myocardium in patients with angina pectoris but normal coronary arteriograms. *Circulation* 1981; **63**: 817–825.

160. Kaski JC, Rosano GMC, Collins P, Nihoyannopoulos P, Maseri A, Poole-Wilson PA. Cardiac syndrome X: clinical characteristics and left ventricular function. Long term follow-up study. *J Am Coll Cardiol* 1995; **25**: 807–814.

161. Rosano GMC, Collins P, Kaski JC, Lindsay DC, Sarrel PM, Poole-Wilson PA. Syndrome X in women is associated with estrogen deficiency. *Eur Heart J* 1995; **16**: 610–614.

162. Rosano GMC, Peters NS, Lefroy DC, et al. 17-beta-estradiol therapy lessens angina in postmenopausal women with syndrome X. *J Am Coll Cardiol* 1996; **28**: 1500–1505.

163. Rosano GMC, Leonardo F, Sarrel PM, Beale CM, De Luca F, Collins P. Cyclical variation in paroxysmal supraventricular tachycardia in women. *Lancet* 1996; **347**: 786–788.

164. Lafferty FW, Fiske ME. Postmenopausal estrogen replacement: a long-term cohort study. *Am J Med* 1994; **97**: 66–77.

165. Nachtigall LE, Nachtigall RH, Nachtigall RD, Beckman EM. Estrogen replacement therapy II: a prospective study in the relationship to carcinoma and cardiovascular and metabolic problems. *Obstet Gynecol* 1979; **54**: 74–79.

166. Psaty BM, Heckbert SR, Atkins D, et al. The risk of myocardial infarction associated with the combined use of estrogens and progestins in postmenopausal women. *Arch Intern Med* 1994; **154**: 1333–1339.

167. Criqui MH, Suarez L, Barrett-Connor E, McPhillips J, Wingard DL, Garland C. Postmenopausal estrogen use and mortality. Results from a prospective study in a defined, homogeneous community. *Am J Epidemiol* 1988; **128**: 606–614.

168. Grodstein F, Stampfer MJ, Manson JE, et al. Postmenopausal estrogen and progestin use and the risk of cardiovascular disease. *N Engl J Med* 1996; **335**: 453–461.

169. Jiang C, Sarrel PM, Lindsay DC, Poole-Wilson PA, Collins P. Progesterone induces endothelium-independent relaxation of rabbit coronary artery in vitro. *Eur J Pharmacol* 1992; **211**: 163–167.

170. Miller VM, Vanhoutte PM. Progesterone and modulation of endothelium-dependent responses in canine coronary arteries. *Am J Physiol* 1991; **261**: R1022–R1027.

171. Williams JK, Honore EK, Washburn SA, Clarkson TB. Effects of hormone replacement therapy on reactivity of atherosclerotic coronary arteries in cynomolgus monkeys. *J Am Coll Cardiol* 1994; **24**: 1757–1761.

172. Rosano GMC, Sarrel PM, Chierchia SL, et al. Medroxy-progesterone (MPA) but not natural progesterone reverses the beneficial effect of estradiol-17β upon exercise induced myocardial ischemia.A double-blind cross-over study. *Circulation* 1996; **94**: I–18.

173. Harbone JB. Phenolic compounds. In: *Phytochemical Methods,* London: Chapman & Hall, 1973: 52–80.

174. Harbone JB. Flavanoids. In: Miller LP (ed.) *Phytochemistry,* New York: Van Nostrand Reinhold, 1973: 344–380.

175. Farnsworth NR, Bingel AS, Cordell GA, Crane FA, Fong HS. Potential value of plants as sources of new antifertility agents II. *J Pharmaceut Sci* 1975; **64**: 717–754.

176. Farmakalidis E, Hathcock JN, Murphy PA. Oestrogenic potency of genistin and daidzin in mice. *Food Chem Toxicol* 1985; **23**: 741–745.

177. Martin PM, Horwitz KB, Ryan DS, McGuire WL. Phytoestrogen interaction with estrogen receptors in human breast cancer cells. *Endocrinology* 1978; **103**: 1860–1867.

178. Kellis JT, Jr., Vickery LE. Inhibition of human estrogen syn-thetase (aromatase) by flavones. *Science* 1984; **225**: 1032–1034.

179. Miksicek RJ. Commonly occurring plant flavonoids have estrogenic activity. *Mol Pharmacol* 1993; **44**: 37–43.

180. Aklyama T, Ishida J, Nakagawa S, et al. Genistein, a specif-ic inhibitor of tyrosine-specific protein kinases. *J Biol Chem* 1987; **262**: 5592–5595.

181. Wijetunge S, Aalkjaer C, Schachter M, Hughes AD. Tyrosine kinase inhibitors block calcium channel currents in vascular smooth muscle cells. *Biochem Biophys Res Commun* 1992; **189**: 1620–1623.

182. Smirnov SV, Aaronson PI. Inhibition of vascular smooth muscle cell K$^+$ currents by tyrosine kinase inhibitors genis-tein and ST 638. *Circ Res* 1995; **76**: 310–316.

183. Nakashima S, Koike T, Nozawa Y. Genistein, a protein tyro-sine kinase inhibitor, inhibits thromboxane A2-mediated human platelet responses. *Mol Pharmacol* 1991; **39**: 475–480.

184. Ozaki Y, Yatomi Y, Jinnai Y, Kume S. Effects of genistein, a tyrosine kinase inhibitor, on platelet functions. Genistein attenuates thrombin-induced Ca^{2+} mobilization in human platelets by affecting polyphosphoninositide turnover. *Biochem Pharmacol* 1993; **46**: 395–403.

185. Sargeant P, Farndale RW, Sage SO. The tyrosine kinase inhibitors methyl 2,5-dihydroxycinnamate and genistein reduce thrombin-evoked tyrosine phosphorylation and Ca^{2+} entry in human platelets. *FEBS Lett* 1993; **315**: 242–246.

186. Asahi M, Yanagi S, Ohta S, et al. Thrombin-induced human platelet aggregation is inhibited by protein-tyrosine kinase inhibitors. *FEBS Lett* 1992; **309**: 10–14.

187. Fotsis T, Pepper M, Adlercreutz H, Fleischmann G, Hase T, Montesano R, Schweigerer L. Genistein, a dietary-derived inhibitor of in vitro angiogenesis. *Proc Natl Acad Sci USA* 1993; **90**: 2690–2694.

188. Honore EK, Williams JK, Anthony MS. Enhancement of coronary vasodilation by soy phytoestrogens and genistein. *Circulation* 1995; **92**: I–349 (abstract).

189. Anthony MS, Clarkson TB, Hughes CL. Plant and mammalian estrogen effects on plasma lipids of female monkeys. *Circulation* 1994; **90**: I–235 (abstract).

190. Anderson JW, Johnstone BM, Cook-Newell ME. Meta-analysis of the effects of soy protein intake on serum lipids. *N Engl J Med* 1995; **333**: 276–282.

191. Adlercreutz H, Markkanen H, Watanabe S. Plasma concentrations of phyto-oestrogens in Japanese men. *Lancet* 1993; **342**: 1209–1210.

192. Adlercreutz H, Hamalainen E, Gorbach S, Goldin B. Dietary phyto-oestrogens and the menopause in Japan. *Lancet* 1992; **339**: 1233.

193. Hertog MG, Feskens EJ, Hollman PC, Katan MB, Kromhout D. Dietary antioxidant flavonoids and risk of coronary heart disease: the Zutphen Elderly Study. *Lancet* 1993; **342**: 1007–1011.

194. Hertog MG, Kromhout D, Aravanis C, et al. Flavonoid intake and long-term risk of coronary heart disease and cancer in the seven countries study. *Arch Intern Med* 1995; **155**: 381–386.

195. Phillips GB, Pinkernell BH, Jing TY. The association of hypotestosteronemia with coronary artery disease in men. *Arterioscler Thromb* 1994; **14**: 701–706.

196. Nordoy A, Aakvaag A, Thelle D. Sex hormones and high density lipoproteins in healthy males. *Atherosclerosis* 1979; **34**: 431–436.

197. Heller RF, Miller NE, Lewis B, et al. Associations between sex hormones, thyroid hormones and lipoproteins. *Clin Sci* 1981; **61**: 649–651.

198. Gutai J, LaPorte R, Kuller L, Dai W, Falvo-Gerard L, Caggiula A. Plasma testosterone, high density lipoprotein cholesterol and other lipoprotein fractions. *Am J Cardiol* 1981; **48**: 897–902.

199. Bagatell CJ, Heiman JR, Matsumoto AM, Rivier JE, Bremner WJ. Metabolic and behavioral effects of high dose, exogenous testosterone in healthy men. *J Clin Endocrinol Metab* 1994; **79**: 561–567.

200. Adams MR, Williams JK, Kaplan JR. Effects of androgens on coronary artery atherosclerosis and atherosclerosis-related impairment of vascular responsiveness. *Arterioscler Thromb Vasc Biol* 1995; **15**: 562–570.

201. Yang XC, Jing TY, Resnick LM, Phillips GB. Relation of hemostatic risk factors to other risk factors for coronary heart disease. *Arterioscler Thromb Vasc Biol* 1993; **13**: 467–471.

202. Caron P, Bennet A, Camare R, Louvet JP, Boneu S, Sie P. Plasminogen activator inhibitor in plasma is related to testosterone in men. *Metabolism* 1989; **38**: 1010–1015.

203. Heller RF, Meade TW, Haines AP, Stirling Y, Miller NE, Lewis B. Inter-relationships between factor VII, serum testosterone and plasma lipoproteins. *Thromb Res* 1982; **28**: 423–425.

204. Bonithon-Kopp C, Scarabin PY, Bara L, Castanier M, Jacqueson A, Roger M. Relationship between sex hormones and haemostatic factors in healthy middle-aged men. *Atherosclerosis* 1988; **71**: 71–76.

205. Matsuda K, Ruff A, Morinelli TA, Mathur RS, Halushka PV. Testosterone increases thromboxane A2 receptor density and responsiveness in rat aortas and platelets. *Am J Physiol* 1994; **267**: H887–H893.

206. Yue P, Chatterjee K, Beale C, Poole-Wilson PA, Collins P. Testosterone relaxes rabbit coronary arteries and aorta. *Circulation* 1995; **91**: 1154–1160.

207. Chou TM, Sudhir K, Hutchison SJ, Ko E, Amidon TM, Collins P, Chatterjee K. Testosterone induces dilation of canine coronary conductance and resistance arteries in vivo. *Circulation* 1996; **94**: 2614–2619.

208. Hamm L. Testosterone propionate in the treatment of angina pectoris. *J Clin Endocrinol* 1942; **2**: 325–328.

209. Walker TC. The use of testosterone propionate and estrogenic substance in the treatment of essential hypertension, angina pectoris and peripheral vascular disease. *J Clin Endocrinol* 1942; **2**: 560–568.

210. Sigler LH, Tulgan J. Treatment of angina pectoris by testosterone propionate. *NY State J Med* 1943; **43**: 1424–1428.

211. Lesser MA. Testosterone propionate therapy in one hundred cases of angina pectoris. *J Clin Endocrinol* 1946; **6**: 549–557.

212. Jaffe MD. Effect of testosterone cypionate on postexercise ST segment depression. *Br Heart J* 1977; **39**: 1217–1222.

Index